Evidence-Based Practice

For Churchill Livingstone

Senior Commissioning Editor Alex Mathieson
Project Manager Jane Shanks

Margaret Pitt 2000

Evidence-Based Practice
A primer for health care professionals

Martin Dawes MD FRCGP
Lecturer in Primary Care, University of Oxford, UK

Philip T. Davies BA(Hons)London MA(California) MLitt(Oxon) MA(Oxon) PhD(California)
Director of Social Sciences, Department for Continuing Education, University of Oxford, UK

Alastair M. Gray BA DPhil
Director, Health Economics Research Centre, University of Oxford, UK

Jonathan Mant MA MBBS MSc MFPHM
Senior Lecturer, Department of Primary Care and General Practice,
University of Birmingham, UK

Kate Seers BSc(Hons) PhD RGN
Head of Research, RCN Institute, Oxford, UK

Robin Snowball BA(Hons) RMN PhD Dip Lib Inf Stud PGCE(Post-Compulsory)
User Education Manager, Cairns Library, John Radcliffe Hospital, Oxford, UK

Foreword by
Professor Alison Kitson RN BSc(Hons) DPhil FRCN
Director, Royal College of Nursing Institute, UK

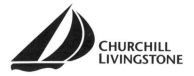

CHURCHILL
LIVINGSTONE

EDINBURGH LONDON NEW YORK PHILADELPHIA ST LOUIS SYDNEY TORONTO 1999

CHURCHILL LIVINGSTONE
An imprint of Harcourt Publishers Limited

© Harcourt Publishers Limited 1999

 is a registered trademark of Harcourt Publishers Limited

The right of Martin Dawes, Philip Davies, Alastair Gray, Jonathan Mant,
Kate Seers and Robin Snowball to be identified as authors of this work
has been asserted by them in accordance with the Copyright, Designs and
Patents Act 1988

First published 1999

0 443 06126 2

British Library Cataloguing in Publication Data
A catalogue record for this book is available from the British Library

Library of Congress Cataloging in Publication Data
A catalog record for this book is available from the Library of Congress

Note
Medical knowledge is constantly changing. As new information becomes
available, changes in treatment, procedures, equipment and the use of
drugs become necessary. The editors/authors/contributors and the
publishers have, as far as it is possible, taken care to ensure that the
information given in this text is accurate and up-to-date. However,
readers are strongly advised to confirm that the information, especially
with regard to drug usage, complies with the latest legislation and
standards of practice.

The
Publisher's
policy is to use
paper manufactured
from sustainable forests

Printed in China

Contents

Foreword

Perhaps the most important skill for any health care professional to master in their career is the ability to recognise and handle clinical uncertainty: uncertainty, as it is manifested in the range of unpredictable and often untimely conditions presented by our patients in wards, outpatients, and in the consulting room; but also uncertainty about one's own skill, expertise and knowledge base.

The ongoing tension between certainty over uncertainty is the driving force of the evidence-based practice movement. Its central philosophy is one of never taking for granted one's own practice, and by using a structured, problem-based approach each practitioner can logically manoeuvre their way through the obstacle race of clinical decision making.

The rigour and discipline of searching for and assessing evidence as outlined in this book is commendable. Its relevance to everyday practice is obvious and its reassuring message is one that each of us needs to understand more fully. It is foolhardy to argue against the rectitude of evidence-based practice approaches and yet paradoxically the greatest risk is that by deriving evidence in this way we may be lulled into a false confidence of clinical certainty!

All each of us can hope for is that we have applied the best available evidence to our care. This publication is a timely aid to help us and reflects the first steps of an ongoing, life-long journey.

Preface

Evidence-based practice is the acknowledgement of uncertainty followed by the seeking, appraising and implementation of new knowledge. It enables clinicians to openly accept that there may be different, and possibly more effective, methods of care than those they are currently employing. No longer can we rely on the information that we were taught as undergraduates to be an adequate source of clinical knowledge for our professional career. Attendance at postgraduate educational events and reading our professional journals are no longer sufficient to keep us aware of all the new developments in practice. To gain this knowledge we need to accept that there are questions we have to ask about our practice. Having posed a number of questions, we should seek answers to the most important, appraise the quality of the resulting evidence and, if appropriate, implement change in response to that new knowledge.

To help that process, this book has been written for health-care professionals interested in evidence-based practice. Whether you are a total novice, or have some experience of searching and appraisal, this book will take you through the concepts, processes and applications of evidence-based practice.

The book has come about as a result of the five authors being involved in setting up and teaching on a Master's degree programme on Evidence-Based Health Care (EBHC). The programme is run for graduates and is based at the University of Oxford. Although other books on various aspects of evidence-based medicine are available, we felt there was a need for an overall text that explores evidence-based practice not only in breadth but also in depth.

We have put together the information that is used on the EBHC course in a format that we hope you will find easy to read and understand. The book, then, is largely a 'how to do it' manual for evidence-based practice. It will take you through the whole process from formulating a question to assessing cost-effectiveness. Evidence-based practice is partly a philosophy, partly a skill and partly the knowledge about, and application of, a set of tools. We have tried to address all these three areas within this book. The major philosophy is one of never taking for granted your own practice.

The beginning of the book helps you phrase those uncertainties into answerable questions and then guides you to the best sources for that information. This will help you direct your searches at the sources of information most likely to yield success and shorten the time of your enquiry.

The next section deals with the evaluation of the quality of that information. Is it really reliable enough for you to change your practice? Next comes more detailed evaluation of the specific types of question. These range from questions about diagnosis and treatment to economic evaluation and qualitative issues. There are guides on how to critically appraise published articles and other types of research. Throughout the book we have used examples that relate to those working at the front line of practice. We teach mixed groups of health-care professionals on the Master's degree programme. They come from all professions working in the health service in the UK and from abroad. We have found that this mix is extremely powerful in enhancing teaching and so have had that audience in mind when writing this book. This is no ivory-towered approach but something we hope you will find practical and useful in your future practice.

Evidence-based practice is not an academic exercise. It is an approach that will lead, ultimately, to an improvement in care but this can only happen if, following the evaluation of the evidence, you change your practice. To further that aim, we have included a section on changing practice as well as monitoring it. Finally, we recognise that as evidence-based practice spreads, more people will be teaching the principles and practice of this approach. We hope that you may pass on some of your newly acquired skills from reading this book, so we have included a chapter on teaching some of the principles of evidence-based practice.

The author should like to thank David Sackett and Muir Gray whose enthusiasm and assistance lay behind the development of the EBHC course at Oxford and this book. In addition, the author should like to thank Geoffrey Thomas, Godfrey Fowler and Martin Vessey for their help.

Oxford, 1999   M.D.

Abbreviations

ARR	absolute risk reduction
CER	control event rate
CI	confidence interval
CME	continuing medical education
EBHC	evidence-based health care
EER	experimental event rate
MeSH	medical subject heading
NNT	numbers needed to treat
PBL	problem-based learning
QALY	quality-adjusted life-year
RCT	randomised controlled trial
ROC	receiver-operating characteristic
RR	relative risk
RRR	relative reduction in risk
SD	standard deviation
SE	standard error
WMD	weighted mean difference
GP	general practitioner

Evidence-based practice

Martin Dawes

But thou art too fine in thy evidence; therefore stand aside.

All's Well That Ends Well. Shakespeare

CLINICAL OVERLOAD

In the last 10 years we have seen the rapid expansion of information about the practice of health care. The number of papers being written, the number of journals being published and the number of postgraduate presentations have all been rising steadily. This increase in information should have resulted in two changes. Our knowledge should be greater and our practice should be more effective. However, at the same time as this increase in information, we have been faced with a greater demand from patients as well as many politically determined structural changes in the health care system.

Our clinical responsibilities can seem overwhelming and we may feel that it is hard enough to stand still let alone question our practice. During our work we often feel under so much pressure that we have scarce time to consider our practice more deeply. When we do question what we do, it is difficult to find time to seek an answer to that question. This is the crux of evidence-based practice. The aim is to use time available to its maximum potential by answering some of these questions to the best of our abilities. By doing this we are increasing knowledge but, more importantly, we are likely to change practice. This change is also likely to occur in an area of practice relevant and important to us as practitioners.

INFORMATION NEED

We usually see an overwhelming number of patients during the week. During each of the sessions or clinics several questions may arise concerning diagnosis, prognosis, treatment and general care. It is therefore quite possible for a practitioner to make many thousands of clinical decisions a year. When asked, general practitioners say that they generate on average two questions per three patients. 40% of the questions were factual (e.g. what dose), 43% were concerned with medical opinion and

17% were non-medical. One-third of these questions are answered at the time of clinical contact. On average, the clinician is left with four unanswered questions per surgery or clinic (Covell et al 1985). We say that we get the answers to these questions mostly from printed sources but, when observed, we tend to get them from colleagues. Much of this information may be completely up to date and accurate but there is no way of ensuring that this is indeed the case.

Evidence for our practice has been gathered over our professional lifetime. This will be from many sources and will depend on how long we have been in practice. The longer we have been practising the more likely our evidence will be based on experience or information from colleagues. In addition there will be evidence from textbooks and postgraduate lectures.

KEEPING UP TO DATE

Practitioners who, to keep up to date, regularly read their professional journal and consult passages in a current textbook as well as attending an occasional postgraduate lecture will only see a very small fraction of the available literature. Only a few of the important studies and relevant evidence concerning common practice problems are published in such journals or textbooks.

To read everything that we need to practise efficiently we would have to read many journals. For those working in primary and public health care the problem is worse than for those working in secondary care. We may deal with diseases seen as the domain of all the hospital specialties within the course of 1 day. A typical clinic or surgery may include the following conditions: migraine, hypertension, diabetes, pregnancy, leg ulcer, dementia, hernia, otitis media, depression, psoriasis and heart failure. Luckily we do not see *all* these conditions in one patient – however, we often see several of them in one patient! To keep up to date therefore would mean reading all the key journals relating to the various specialties, which might mean, for example, that you needed to cover 30 journals a week. There is absolutely no way that can be achieved. Yet if you want to know the effective surgical treatment for ingrown toe nail, then the randomised control trials are not published in the British Medical Journal or Nursing Times but are all (bar one) to be found in surgical journals.

WHAT IS EVIDENCE-BASED PRACTICE?

It is against this background of information need and clinical overload and the general feeling of helplessness that evidence-based practice can offer some help. In its most basic definition it aims to provide the best possible evidence at the point of clinical (or management) contact. This book will outline how that can be achieved whilst realising the practical constraints of working in a health service. It aims at ensuring that decisions are made on evidence that has been appraised critically and presented in understandable terms rather than research jargon.

To practise evidence-based practice you need to ask questions about the care; for example 'Is this treatment effective?' The next step is to break that question down into something that is answerable. The reformulated question might then contain information about the disease and the patient. The evidence answering your question would be identified and appraised and finally the evidence put into practice.

It has been suggested that evidence for more than a tiny fraction of the decisions made cannot possibly be available. 10 years ago this may have been a legitimate argument but today it is no longer the case. There is now a wide, published database of information on many aspects of health care. This information is often published in journals with small readerships and may rarely be seen. Yet the information may be extremely important. Other evidence may be published and widely disseminated but we may be too busy to read it. More commonly we are trying to read too much too quickly and so fail to realise the importance of certain information. Finally, even if we did see an important article, how would we remember it and apply it in our practice?

EVIDENCE

To answer specific health-care questions there are some optimal types of research. An example is the study of rare side effects from a drug, for example, thrombosis and the combined oral contraceptive pill. As the numbers required to observe the potential side effects are very large, a sizeable cohort (i.e. recruitment of several thousand individuals followed for some years) will be needed. An alternative, cheaper and therefore more achievable study is the case control study. This form of study looks backwards at the factors affecting those who have had events, and those who are 'matched controls' (matched by age and sex and any other important variables).

The ideal, though not always possible, way to evaluate a treatment is to randomly allocate the experimental treatment or a placebo to patients (after gaining their permission). Ideally the person giving the treatment, having the treatment, and evaluating the clinical effect should not know which treatment is being used. At the end of treatment the outcome is assessed in the two groups. The number of these randomised controlled trials (RCTs) is now huge (Dickersin et al 1994), and those indexed on electronic databases under the umbrella of 'primary care', although still relatively small when compared to hospital medicine, have increased 5-fold since 1986 (Silagy & Jewell 1994). Moreover, answers to many common primary care questions are found in research performed and published outside primary care (Silagy 1993). Thus, a computer search identified 9 randomised trials on the treatment of ingrown toe nails, 38 on atopic dermatitis, and 11 on the treatment of glue ear, but only one (glue ear) was published in a primary care journal.

Similar increases in the publication of therapeutic trials conducted by professions allied to medicine are also seen (Cullum 1997). More evidence about the cause and prognosis of diseases is also being published. There is also an increase in publications of qualitative research on the impact of disease and treatment on people as individuals.

Much high quality, relevant evidence is already there, but it remains invisible to most practitioners, even to those who have the opportunity to keep up with the mainstream journals. Having argued that the evidence is available, another barrier is that practitioners find it difficult to find the time to track it down. The move towards a more evidence-based practice does not require that every practitioner tracks down evidence on every question or appraises all the evidence.

CRITICAL APPRAISAL

Unfortunately we cannot just accept that most papers published by reputable journals are of sufficient quality for us to believe them. Journals rely on peer review by volunteers who are often given a short time to comment on several papers. During this process there is a decision that has to be made not only about the quality of the paper but also about its potential importance. If the information is very important or topical, it may override the flaws in the research process. This clearly is not a satisfactory outcome but is still sometimes the case.

A piece of research may have a very meaningful outcome suggesting that one particular form of practice is better than another. However, there may be flaws in the way the research was performed. These flaws may occur anywhere along the process and not only, as some may assume, in the statistical analysis. Critical appraisal is important to examine the rigour with which a study was conducted, and thus the amount of confidence you can place in the findings.

For example, a study may not have found out what happened to every one of the patients involved (follow-up). This is often the case, but in some studies the rate of follow-up may be as low as 60%. The authors may not know what happened to more than one-third of patients and it may be that those patients not followed up had a different outcome to those who were described in the paper. This is one example of a methodological weakness detected by critical appraisal. Although the process is straightforward, it can take some time and if a piece of research has been through this process already, then this is very helpful.

SHORT CUTS

Some of the evidence for answering clinical questions in public health or primary care already has been tracked down, critically appraised, and packaged in easily accessible forms (Box 1.1). The format of these publications differs in length and style but the publications have one common feature. The available material has all been through a rigorous, critical appraisal. The appraisal has addressed the issues of quality that are described later on.

Box 1.1   Sources of evidence-based publications

- The Evidence Based Medicine Journal and the ACP Journal Club
- ACP Journal Club on Disk. Haynes R B (ed). American College of Physicians, Philadelphia, Serial software for PC or Macintosh
- Evidence Based Medicine published by the British Medical Journal
- Bandolier. Hayward Medical Communications, Rosemary House, Lanwades Park, Kentford, Near Newmarket, Suffolk CB8 7PW
- Effectiveness Matters and Effective Health Care bulletins
- NHS Centre for Reviews and Dissemination (CRD), University of York, York YO1 5DD
- The Cochrane Library, Update Software Ltd, Summertown Pavilion, Middle Way, Oxford OX2 7LG. Web-site: http://www.cochrane.co.uk
- Evidence Based Health Policy and Management. Churchill Livingstone, Robert Stevenson House, 1–3 Baxter's Place, Leith Walk, Edinburgh EH1 3AF

To use journals that have filtered positively for good quality research information is a useful mechanism for general reading. The articles are often rewritten by these secondary journals in short formats. Many of these single-page abstracts and commentaries relate to public health and primary care issues. Because only about 2% of the clinical articles in the 50 journals screened for these publications pass both scientific and clinical criteria, the reading time now required to keep up with important clinical advances is a smaller, more feasible fraction of its former, unmanageable magnitude.

A rapidly expanding resource is the Cochrane Library of Systematic Reviews. This resource, already available on computer diskette and compact disc, contains extensively and methodically searched reviews of randomised trials on the clinical and economic effects of health care, and already has become a practical resource for practitioners in all fields of patient care.

LIBRARIES

Many issues in health care have not gone through this careful assembly and appraisal, and reliance on non-evidence-based reviews is risky. To address this, practitioners must spend the time required to find the evidence. The amount of time for searching will vary with each individual question, but the practitioner who can find 1 hour a week in which to search and read will start to make huge strides. Often the solution is found in searching the electronic publications described above, with the additional bonus of obviating the need to carry out the tasks of critical appraisal. But when this approach is unsuccessful, the next stage involves an electronic search of the literature, either on one's own or with the assistance of a librarian. Health libraries are very much more aware of the needs of practitioners and most can receive requests for papers by telephone and fax them to the practitioner the same day. In most searches, the associated abstracts can be downloaded, and often provide sufficient information to determine the methodological approach of the research, its clinical relevance and application (McKibbon & Walker-Dilks 1994a, McKibbon & Walker-Dilks 1994b, McKibbon & Walker-Dilks 1994c, Walker-Dilks et al 1994).

The latest innovation is the National Electronic Library for Health. This will be a real building but also a virtual library with access to as many sources of information as possible. With real librarians to e-mail for help, it will act as a national resource for knowledge.

COURSES ON SEARCHING AND APPRAISAL

Practitioners often feel that they lack the necessary skills and experience to critically appraise the evidence and determine its applicability within their locality. The experience we have gained in teaching these skills has led to this book. We feel that many of the skills can be developed by practice using various specific skills outlined here. However, learning to appraise with others can be a more effective way of gaining these skills.

There is no question that being taught how to search by an experienced librarian is far more efficient than trying to practise it oneself with minimum instruction. Therefore, to build on the knowledge gained from reading this book we also recommend attendance at one of the many courses on evidence-based health care. Guidelines for critical appraisal are being disseminated widely following these courses. In recognition of the importance of these skills, the examination for the UK Royal College of General Practitioners has for several years included a section requiring the critical appraisal of a clinical article.

STORING AND RETRIEVING EVIDENCE

The final hurdle facing a practitioner is that relevant evidence cannot be recalled during the consultation when the answers are required. Even if successful in solving all the foregoing, the practitioner faces the challenge of storing the results of searches and critical appraisals in ways that can be readily accessed for future use. Setting search results aside for later filing and organisation is likely to be a recipe for frustration and failure. With computers on the desks of growing numbers of practitioners or hand-held electronic organisers, the potential exists for keeping these results within easy reach, especially the evidence needed to assist the most frequent questions and decisions.

The future is here now; it just is not evenly distributed yet! And even with these solutions, there remain too many questions for an individual practitioner to answer. But help is on the way. With the growing number of practitioners learning how to search and critically appraise, the opportunities for progress are rapidly increasing. For example, in the UK, primary care researchers, trainers of family practitioners and postgraduate tutors cover the whole country are promoting a critical approach to primary care practice and research. As these and similar groups share the tasks of searching for and appraising evidence, they can collate their critical appraisals electronically in agreed formats. These can be assembled together to make a database of answered questions. The forthcoming National Electronic Library for Health will act as a coordinator for the delivery of this and other formats of information and evidence to all areas of the Health Service.

REFERENCES

Covell D, Uman G, Manning P 1985 Information needs in office practice: are they being met? Annals of Internal Medicine 103:596–599
Cullum N 1997 Identification and analysis of randomised control trials in nursing: preliminary study. Quality in Health Care 6
Dickersin K, Scherer R, Lefebvre C 1994 Identifying relevant studies for systematic reviews. British Medical Journal 309:1286–1291
McKibbon K A, Walker-Dilks C 1994a Beyond ACP Journal Club: how to harness MEDLINE for diagnostic problems [editorial]. ACP Journal Club 121(Suppl 2):A10–12
McKibbon K, Walker-Dilks C 1994b Beyond ACP Journal Club: how to harness MEDLINE for therapy problems [editorial]. ACP Journal Club 121 (Suppl 1):A10–12
McKibbon K, Walker-Dilks C 1994c Beyond ACP Journal Club: how to harness MEDLINE to solve clinical problems [editorial]. ACP Journal Club 120(Suppl 2):A10–12
Silagy C 1993 Developing a register of randomised controlled trials in primary care. British Medical Journal 306:897–900
Silagy C, Jewell D 1994 Review of 39 years of randomized controlled trials in the British Journal of General Practice. British Journal of General Practice 44:359–363
Walker-Dilks C, McKibbon K, Haynes R 1994 Beyond ACP Journal Club: how to harness MEDLINE for etiology problems [editorial]. ACP Journal Club 121:A10–11

2

Formulating a question

Martin Dawes

Sitting at your desk one afternoon with the sun coming through the window, your mind drifts off to the holiday you have just returned from. Suddenly your patient shuffles noisily and you are brought back to the real world. This daydream may have only taken a few seconds but provides you with the energy to continue the endless stream of work.

The amount of work that we all have to complete is sometimes over-whelming and we forget to ask what we are doing. The patient presents, you listen to the history, make an examination and, where appropriate, order some tests or start some therapy. Nothing wrong with that except: have you had time to think about alternatives? Is there a better way to listen to the history? Are the examinations appropriate and what is their clinical significance? What might be the meaning of the diagnostic tests, and which treatments are most effective for this condition? Or is it all too much and should you just carry on with occasional daydreams?

Consider a different daydream, one that would take the same length of time. Instead of drifting back to that holiday, ask yourself: what are the options here? Is this ritualistic examination of the chest of any value? Is this antibiotic going to affect outcome? Is this bandage the most effective? This questioning atti-tude is what makes us good professionals. Are we doing the **right** things, and if so are they being done in the **right** way and at the **right** time (Gray 1997)?

The reason we do not usually ask questions is they are so difficult to answer. This was nicely illustrated in *The Hitch Hiker's Guide to the Galaxy* when the super computer gave the answer '42' to the question: 'What does life, the universe and everything mean?' (Adams 1994). The people asking the question were horrified and angry. The computer calmly suggested that instead of panicking they should go back and consider the question and that he would of course help them to do this. This is an extreme example of how a question can be so badly formed that its answer is meaningless.

It is a trap we can easily fall into in practice. I go to see a patient with a leg ulcer at home at the request of the district nurse. The ulcer is chronic, painful and inflamed. What should I do? The instant thought is 'I don't know enough about leg ulcers to carry on the management without some help.' Having heard about evidence-based practice, I decide to ask the question 'What is the best management for leg ulcers?' I give antibiotics to the patient and return home for lunch.

I turn on my computer and use the modem to connect to the British Medical Association 'on-line' Medline Library. I have done this using some software that my son installed for me from a CD-ROM that came with a computer magazine. It is called America On-Line (AOL) and means I can get access to the World Wide Web from home (at a cost!). The modem kicks into action and after 20 seconds my computer screen tells me I am connected and asks me for a password. It then says I can type in my search question. I search on the term 'leg ulcer' and it says there are 3940 articles, the first being about Manuka honey and leg ulcers! I give up and eat my lunch.

I went wrong in two places. First, my search was unstructured. This is dealt with in the next chapter. Second, what was my question? I wanted to know more about leg ulcers, but why? My patient was an 83-year-old woman living alone at home with well-controlled (dietary) diabetes and some moderate heart failure for which she was on diuretic therapy (yes, I know she should have been on an angiotensin-converting enzyme inhibitor but this is the real world!). Using a walking frame she was mobile around the house but rarely got out. Her immediate problem was pain.

I could have gone to a textbook and read thoroughly about leg ulcers but I do not have the time. There are many questions that arise from any consultation and being human we can only deal with those that are most important. In this case it may have been pain.

My question should have focused on the relief of pain caused by leg ulcers. This is the end point of my inquiry. If added to my search on leg ulcer, it would now only show those papers dealing with pain as well as leg ulcers so that I would not be quite so swamped with information. I am really only interested at the moment in my patient who is an 83-year-old woman living alone etc. So my question is really about patients who are elderly and diabetic. I could have just chosen elderly but I felt that the diabetes was probably significant in determining the aetiology and therefore likely to be relevant to the therapy.

My question is now: 'In elderly diabetics with chronic leg ulcers, what is the most effective therapy for removing pain?'

It is becoming better but the middle part is still vague. Perhaps I should enter some of the therapeutic options I know about, antibiotics for example. I need not do this but could carry on searching. If I was uncertain about the therapies, this would be a useful search but quite large. In this case I found 173 articles of which 14 were classified as randomised controlled trials and included such therapies as electromagnetism and nifedipine.

Now I am getting somewhere. By structuring a question, the answer may be found more efficiently. It is therefore important to try to break the question down into several parts (Richardson et al 1995).

1. Patient or problem
2. Intervention

3. Comparison intervention (optional)
4. Outcomes.

PATIENT OR PROBLEM

The first part is to identify the problem or the patient. Health-care problems may not always seem to be about patients! For example, an administrator may want to know whether having acute medical beds in a temporary holding ward next to the Accident and Emergency department is any more efficient than having conventional acute medical wards in the hospital. In this case the question is concerned with the hospital in which the administrator works. Another example is the use of nurses in out-of-hours provision of telephone advice for a medical group. In this situation nurses may be employed in addition to receptionists to filter calls to the doctors providing out-of-hours service within primary care. In this case the 'problem or patient' may be the out-of-hours cooperative.

Make sure at this stage in the question that you are describing the problem or patients that you see. These may be patients within certain specialist settings who would respond differently from those within the community (see Ch. 16). However, if you are too specific at this stage, you may miss some important evidence and there is a balance to be struck between getting evidence about exactly your group of patients and getting *all* the evidence about *all* groups of patients.

INTERVENTION

The intervention is equally important. It may in fact be a postponement of an action such as an operation. In patients with abdominal pain lasting less than 12 hours, does an additional 24-hour delay before referral to hospital alter outcome? Most interventions are more straightforward such as types of dressings, drug therapies or counselling. Alternatively they can be the provision of differing environmental factors such as the décor of waiting rooms or deal with the way in which information is given to patients (Thomas 1987).

Be as specific as possible with the intervention at this stage. You may want to backtrack later if you cannot find any evidence. What regimen of drug therapy are you interested in? If you are working in primary care, then oral methods of drug delivery will be more appropriate than intravenous. Is that therapy going to be the same as you can provide? The way in which we offer treatment to patients varies from both within and between primary and secondary care. The frequency with which we can see patients and alter doses as well as the ability to check serum levels may be different from secondary care, and all these factors may affect outcomes.

The types of interventions may be quite varied and you often have to consider this quite carefully when refining the question. For example, you may have a question about the prognosis or aetiology of a condition. The intervention can be causative factors for aetiological questions. Therefore, you may want to include passive smoking as your intervention when questioning the cause of cancer. Equally you might include certain operations for the investigation of the prognosis of a cancer.

COMPARISON INTERVENTION

Sometimes there is a comparison of the intervention. For example, you might seek papers comparing the use of head lice lotion in children compared with placebo (Vander Stichele et al 1995). Considering whether looking for comparative studies will help when searching for that evidence.

OUTCOMES

Outcome measures are particularly important when considering the question. It is worth spending some time working out exactly what it is you want. In serious diseases it is often easy to concentrate on the mortality and miss the important aspects of morbidity. For example, the use of toxic chemotherapies for cancer may affect both aspects.

STRUCTURING THE QUESTION

Finally, it is useful when developing the question to use a grid (Table 2.1). Initially, I start with the question jotted down on a piece of paper and stuffed in my pocket. When I examine the bits of paper later, I decide which questions I want to spend time exploring. My jottings are usually very unstructured, containing some details about the patient (usually the name so I can enter the result of the search into the patient's notes later) and the condition with something about an intervention. The next step is then to

Table 2.1 Sample grid for structuring questions

Patient or problem	Intervention	Comparison intervention	Outcomes

refine the question. This does take a little time and it is well worth spending a few minutes considering the various possible alternative outcomes or interventions. I write these alternatives down in the grid and then these are used to perform the searches.

Using this process I know I have developed a question that is more likely to result in a significant and useful answer. The objective is for us as clinicians to continue to ask questions. Then we will retain and increase our enthusiasm for one of the most rewarding professions.

REFERENCES

Adams D 1994 Life, the universe, and everything. The hitch hiker's guide to the galaxy, 3. Millennium (Orion), London
Gray J 1997 Doing the right things right. In: Evidence based health-care. Churchill Livingstone, New York, ch 2, p17
Richardson W, Wilson M, Nishikawa J, Hayward R S 1995 The well-built clinical question: a key to evidence-based decisions [editorial]. ACP Journal Club 123:A12–13
Thomas K 1987 General practice consultations: is there any point in being positive? British Medical Journal Clinical Research Edition 294:1200–1202
Vander Stichele R, Dezeure E, Bogaert M 1995 Systematic review of clinical efficacy of topical treatments for head lice. British Medical Journal 311:604–608

3

Finding the evidence: an information skills approach

Robin Snowball

INTRODUCTION

Once we have a clear and structured question, we can work together through a logical process for finding and using the best resources for the main types of question we may ask in our search for *information*. Information-seeking is a central and integral part of the process in which we begin by formulating questions about problematic aspects of complex situations in the real world, in order, ultimately, to make informed decisions or to influence change. More than ever before, we need the skills – new for many of us, but now key skills – to search both *for* and *within* potential information resources of many kinds, and to exploit the 'best' for our particular purposes, effectively and efficiently.

In terms of sheer quantity, there seems to have been an information 'big bang'. Mulrow (1995), for example, tells us that 2 million articles are published annually in some 20 000 'biomedical' journals: a pile of paper some 500 metres high! In addition, information which could serve as good evidence may be buried even deeper, in unpublished studies, or in those undisseminated publications known as 'grey' (Europe) or 'black' (USA) literature. Our electronic new age is radically changing patterns of information recording, dissemination and access, and the resources we must use to locate research-derived information are proliferating in all disciplines and subjects and in a bewildering variety of forms.

All the more reason, then, to take a systematic approach to finding and using the best available information resources for the various types of questions we might ask across health-care practice and research. Using our own structured questions, as described in Chapter 2, we will work through five key questions as a guide:

1. What type of *question* is being asked?
2. What sort of *information* would provide evidence to answer this type of question?
3. What type of *study* would provide such information?
4. What types of *information resources* would give us access to (the results of) such studies?
5. How do we get the *best* out of the resources, to answer each type of question?

In addressing question 4, we will take a brief overview of the main types of current information resource, with examples. In answering question 5, we will look at getting the best out of computer bibliographic databases and finding World Wide Web sites: key resource types. The chapter will close with a summary of the key information skills for finding evidence, and it is followed by a Select List of Information Resources, detailing some 150 current resources, many of which are mentioned in the chapter, indicated by numbers in brackets, for example (35). This is a get-started list, as no such list is ever comprehensive. 'Learning the resources' is a continuing task, for which you can enlist the support of those valuable human resources: your local, specialist, health-care librarians!

Terminology is a minefield. I use '*resources*' to cover the entire range of 'sources' in or from which 'information' may be discovered or constructed, when these exist in any accessible physical form – organisations, web sites, computer databases, journals and printed materials – cutting across the traditional distinction between 'primary' and 'secondary' sources.

'*Information*' includes 'data' (statistics, values, etc.), the raw material from which information (expressed in statements or propositions) may be derived. Since various kinds of information can be *used as* 'evidence,' of varying degrees of strength, appropriate to question type and context, I will not make an essential distinction between 'evidence resources' and 'information resources'.

PUTTING TOGETHER A RESOURCES STRATEGY

Let us now work through our sequence of questions, trying out examples. You will find it makes more sense if you run through the process after formulating your own 'clinical' or structured question, as shown in Chapter 2. Searching, like research, needs the focus of a clear, specific question, however provisional. Of course, a preliminary search can help you formulate or sharpen your question, before you search more thoroughly! Some simple questions – what Richardson & Wilson (1997) call 'background' questions about the basic facts of a disease or a therapy – are not complex enough to have 'parts', and may be answered from basic resources such as textbooks or formularies. But even a 'simple', clinical question, like the leg ulcer question in Chapter 2, may be opened out by using the question structure to clarify and direct the search at the outset. It is here, at the start, that many searches get lost!

Stop now, and formulate your *own* question before you continue!

1. WHAT TYPE OF *QUESTION* IS BEING ASKED?

Richardson et al (1995) in their concise summary of clinical question formulation checklist the main question types to help us formulate questions. We can adapt their categories, adding others as we need them, to help us 'locate' our questions:

- **Clinical findings**: How do we properly gather or soundly interpret (these) clinical findings?
- **Differential diagnosis**: How do we distinguish condition *a* from condition *b*?
- **Diagnostic tests**: How do we select and interpret relevant diagnostic tests for *x*?
- **Therapy**: Is this intervention more effective (in terms of stated outcome/s) than another/others/doing nothing, etc.?
- **Prevention**: How do we screen and reduce the risk of this disease?
- **Prognosis**: What is the likely outcome, course or natural progression, of this condition?
- **Cause/aetiology**: What are the causes of this state of affairs?
- **Cost-effectiveness**: Is intervention *a* more cost-effective than intervention *b*?
- **Harm/risk**: What are the side effects, risks etc. of this intervention? (Does it do more harm than good?)
- **Quality of life**: What will be the quality of life for the patient(s) following (or without) this intervention?

Let's take a question about hormone replacement therapy and its effect on osteoporosis as an example:

Q. In post-menopausal women, does hormone replacement therapy (HRT) prevent osteoporosis?

This may be a therapy question, a prevention question, a risk–benefit question or a cost-effectiveness question: we need to be clear which it is from the start. The therapy question type has served as a model in evidence-based *medicine*, for obvious reasons, but there is a wide range of question types across *health-care* practice and research. A question about the 'quality of life' of those receiving treatment is a more complex 'qualitative' question type. A question about prostate cancer screening might be a cost-effectiveness question, a screening-effectiveness question or a prevention question. If we have more than one question or question type, we must distinguish between them, since each may require different kinds of information for evidence, and, possibly, different types of resources. We may even need a different search approach *within* resources, as we shall see when we look at searching computer databases effectively.

Stop now, and decide, however provisionally, a fundamental *question type* for your question.

2. WHAT SORT OF *INFORMATION* WOULD PROVIDE EVIDENCE TO ANSWER THIS TYPE OF QUESTION?

We next need to be able to recognise the types of information which may be used as evidence, from the strongest to the weakest, appropriate to our question type. The type of information we would use as the strongest evidence for a therapy question is not the same as for a question about cost-effectiveness or prognosis, or for 'qualitative' issues such as consumer satisfaction or quality of life. So we may not find it in the same resources. Other chapters discuss in detail the types of evi-dence required for these and other question types: our concern is with clearly identifying the types of information resources appropriate to them.

The best evidence for a therapy question will be provided by information about defined outcomes resulting from use of the therapy in one group of patients, compared with its non-use in another. This will be stronger as systematic bias is decreased by random allocation, blinding, etc. (see Ch. 5). The next best evidence might be provided by information about the effects in a certain population, then about the effects in an individual, and so on down the evidence 'pyramid' – from strongest to weakest evidence – for this question type. Health economics questions (Chs 10 and 15) require a complex combination of infor-mation on effectiveness and cost. For prognosis questions, the best evidence might be provided by information about survival rates over specified times, or descriptions of the course of the disease, in a specified population, with the weakest evidence from individual case studies.

Issues of *quantitative* and *qualitative* evidence (see Ch. 11, and Popay & Williams 1998) arise here. What sort of *information* might serve as the best evidence for quality-of-life questions? For some types of question, including some therapy questions, qualitative factors which are difficult or impossible to quantify are involved. Values, cultural perceptions or other types of 'soft' complexity make generalisation between groups or populations difficult or inappropriate, yet 'evidence' is needed for decision-making. What sort of information would provide evidence to answer questions such as: 'What forms of terminal care interventions best meet the psychological needs of individuals with life-threatening diseases?' or to address questions where even definitions are contested, such as 'How are crises of gender identity in adolescents most effectively resolved?'

So, draft your evidence 'pyramid' of the type of information which would provide the 'best' or strongest evidence down to that which would provide the weakest, most applicable to *your* type of question – filling in knowledge gaps from other chapters of this book.

3. WHAT TYPE OF *STUDY* WOULD PROVIDE SUCH INFORMATION?

We must next ask what types of study or investigation will provide the information we can use as evidence, from the strongest to the weakest, for each particular type of question. We usually answer this and the previous question simultaneously, but it may help to isolate the logically prior question about types of information to use as evidence first, opening up new perspectives for some, especially qualitative, question types. The understandable dominance of the (mainly medical) therapy model may lead us to believe that information from randomised controlled trials (RCTs) or from systematic reviews of RCTs is the best, even the only admissible, evidence for *all* types of question, and that if we cannot find these, we have no evidence! A well-conducted RCT should provide the information we can use as evidence for therapy effectiveness questions, such as the use of antibiotics to treat leg ulcers. A systematic review of such trials, including the statistical form of systematic review known as meta-analysis, should provide even sounder evidence. (For practical purposes, a properly evidence-based clinical practice guideline – see Ch. 12 – might summarise the best evidence for making rapid clinical decisions.) If these are unavailable, we would look for non-randomised clinical trials, and so on 'down' the pyramid of evidence studies for this type of question. If there are no trials, perhaps for a rare condition, we may find only case reports.

Toward the base of the evidence pyramid for therapy, we might have to cite the opinion of respected and experienced authorities, or 'anecdotal' evidence (but see Enkin & Jadad 1988). For a prognosis question, a cohort study might provide the best evidence; for risk or harm questions, case-control studies might provide the best evidence currently available. For our terminal care question – and for those many 'health interventions ... which are not readily amenable to rigorous experimental research design' (Popay & Williams, 1998:32) – controlled trials may be all but impossible to set up, for many reasons, including ethical ones.

It may be impossible to easily or usefully quantify key factors, and individual, group, cultural or other contextual differences might make comparison or generalisation difficult. So qualitative research may provide information for complex health policy decisions: Popay & Williams (1998) cite as an example Goffman's classic work (1961) on institutionalisation in mental hospitals, which greatly influenced national policy change. For terminal care, we might search for studies describing the outcomes of specific care strategies for the dying in various contexts, but information on cultural practices and beliefs, 'insider' phenomenological descriptions of the experience of terminal illness, and so on – from a very wide range of information resources – may provide the best evidence available for making informed decisions.

So we need to be clear about the type of *information* we really need, and the types of studies which would generate it, in order to find the best information resources, and even to tailor specific search strategies for using those resources most effectively.

What types of study or investigation would yield the information which would provide the best evidence – from strongest to weakest – appropriate to *your* question type?

List them now!

4. WHAT TYPES OF *RESOURCES* WOULD GIVE US ACCESS TO (THE RESULTS OF) SUCH STUDIES?

First, let us recapitulate what we have established, however provisionally, by this stage. These simple strands will form our golden thread for beginning to explore the global labyrinth of resources:

- the detailed, specific question we want to answer
- the real 'purpose' of our question expressed as a question type
- the 'best' types of evidence to answer different types of question
- the types of study or investigation that would provide such evidence.

The sheer variety of resources in our rapidly expanding universe of information seems alarming, but now we can begin to map *types of study* to the main *types of resource* in which information may be found. We can also include those vital types of resource which refer us to those resources which actually hold the information. This is the traditional distinction between '*primary*' sources in which original studies are published, and '*secondary*' sources which refer to or give 'bibliographical' access in the form of references to material in primary sources. (This is now a distinction of function rather than form: many journals fulfil both functions, and full-text databases deliver original publications in full.)

We can now take a brief and simplified overview of the main current *types* of information resource, and then look at them in table form, to link them to types of studies. We can then go to our Select List of Information Resources, and begin searching for specific resources.

First of all, many original studies are written up, but not published (i.e. publicly issued). It has been suggested (Stern & Simes 1997) that those with inconclusive or negative conclusions are more likely to be rejected by those who peer review articles for publication in journals. A 'publication bias' toward 'positive' conclusions may thus result, so it may be important to trace unpublished work, as systematic reviewers do, to get a more complete picture of work that has been done. So directories or databases of research and trials registers are major types of resource, increasingly available.

Second, many studies are published, but are not publicised or made widely available. These include valuable resources such as theses and dissertations, as well as circulars, reports and other material produced by the health service and other organisations. This 'grey' literature may contain the very information we need, but it is notoriously difficult to trace or obtain. Indexes or databases of theses, dissertations and other 'grey' literature are valuable tools.

Third, studies which *do* get published may appear in primary peer-reviewed journals. In addition to the annually published 2 million articles in the 20 000 journals referred to by Mulrow (1995), there are thousands more general and specialist journals in subjects which may be relevant to health-care questions, such as social sciences, education or psychology. This tidal wave of information has created an urgent need for authoritative, comprehensive and accessible reviews of the large numbers of original studies in which vital information may still be 'buried'. Many general reviews do not meet the criteria for 'systematic' review, but are 'subjective, scientifically unsound and inefficient' (Mulrow 1987). Good systematic reviews (see Oxman 1995 for a checklist of criteria) are now recognised as of critical importance, and so review journals have begun to appear. In addition, 'secondary' journals now alert us to material in primary journals that may be of special significance in clinical decision-making, along with comments or critical appraisal. Many primary journals now contain sections for this very useful function. Journals are increasingly accessible on the World Wide Web: some offer contents lists or references, while others offer full-text articles; some are subscription-based, perhaps offering free selections, while others are free of charge.

The history of the scientific and professional journal, which began as a 'journal' or diary passed among small groups of scientists in mid-17th century England and France, is fascinating. Without such information transfer, scientific and technical progress as we know it would have been impossible. (For one view of the future, see Smith 1991.) It is still our major primary resource, which explains the crucial importance of our major *secondary* resources: printed bibliographic indexes and computer bibliographic databases. These give us swift access to the contents of journals and other forms of primary literature published worldwide. They range, as do journals, from the general to the super-specialised. They are called 'bibliographic' because they provide references (often with abstracts) to original studies and to reviews of original studies. Databases which deliver full-text articles rather than bibliographic references are emerging, such as ExtraMed, and Health CD. Newer databases such as the Cochrane Library deliver full text on systematic reviews, and databases of guidelines are starting to appear in an attempt to cope with the explosion of original studies published as journal articles. Many journals are not covered by standard databases, however, and the true contents of original articles from those that do appear may not be properly described by author abstracts or by indexers. These are problems which systematic reviewers address by 'hand searching' key journals, but any of us might miss vital information because of them.

Bibliographical databases appear in many formats. The invention of the portable, high-capacity compact disk (CD-ROM) enabled huge databases of bibliographical records, previously produced as printed indexes, to be made accessible via search software on a personal computer (PC) or small network. Databases are now also increasingly Internet- or Web-accessible, free of charge or subscription-based; access to the whole database, search features, free print or download options and transmission time may all, however, vary between providers.

As well as journals – a slow form of communication by modern standards – valuable information now appears in bulletins, such as effectiveness bulletins, and in newsletters, all in a variety of formats, printed and Web-accessible, targeted at specific interest groups or subjects.

Finally, reports form a growing body of literature. Formally published reports can be found via databases, web sites or library catalogues – but all too many remain distinctly 'grey'.

And now, cutting across all these categories, comes the Internet. World Wide Web sites provide increasing access to both primary and secondary resources: to databases, journals, studies, reviews, newsletters, bulletins, project groups, organisations, discussion groups, libraries and individuals. The information universe is fragmenting fast: there is no central resource in which 'everything' can be found on anything at all!

Table 3.1 attempts a simplified overview of the main types of resources.

Column 1 lists the main 'publication types' (an ambiguous term, but MEDLINE-sanctioned at least!) – the types of 'study' discussed in the previous section.

Column 2 lists the main types of *primary* resource in which such studies are published. The numbers in brackets link them to the publication types of Column 1.

Column 3 lists the main types of *secondary* resource: those which refer us to the main primary resources of Column 2, to which they are linked by the capital letters in brackets.

The Select List of Information Resources on pages **34–46** has numbered entries: examples of entries from the Select List appear in Columns 2 and 3, so you can browse between Table 3.1 and the Select List.

5. HOW DO WE GET THE BEST OUT OF THE RESOURCES, TO ANSWER EACH TYPE OF QUESTION?

We need to be able to exploit information resources effectively, not missing too much of importance, nor getting overwhelmed by 'rubbish'. We must exploit the trade-off between:

1. **comprehensiveness**: finding everything of any relevance at all – but with higher likelihood of retrieving 'rubbish:' a high sensitivity/low specificity search, and
2. **selectivity**: finding only the most highly relevant material – but with a higher likelihood of missing valuable material: a low sensitivity/high specificity search.

Table 3.1   Main types of primary and secondary resources available to researchers

Types of 'publication'	Primary resources	Secondary resources
1. **Clinical guidelines** 'Evidence-based'	A. **Primary journals** These cover publication types 1–5 in column 1. Examples are 47,48,49, 58,59,61–64 in Select List of information Resources.	**Secondary journals** These cover primary resources A in column 2. Examples are 46,50,52–56,60 in Select List of Information Resources.
2. **Systematic reviews** (incl. meta-analyses)		
3. **Reviews**		**Databases/indexes:**
4. **Original studies** a. RCTs b. controlled trials c. clinical trials d. case-control studies e. cohort studies f. prospective studies g. cross-sectional studies h. comparative studies i. longitudinal studies j. population studies k. retrospective studies l. surveys m. qualitative studies	B. **Trials and research registers** These cover 4a–c. Examples are 17,36,38,41 C. **Effectiveness bulletins** These cover 2, 4a–c. Examples are 65,68,69,71,73. D. **Bulletins and newsletters** These cover 1–4, projects, news, etc. Examples are 65–75.	• bibliographical databases cover A,B,C,E,F,G in column 2 • full-text databases are primary resources for column 1 items — general health-care databases e.g. 9,11,15,23,35 — subject or discipline databases e.g. 2,4,5,12,14,25, 39,45 — social aspects of health care e.g. 6,8,27,41,43,44 — economic aspects e.g. 13,22,29,37 — reviews e.g. 7,13,17,19 — 'grey' literature e.g. 17,21,31,33,43 — guidelines e.g. 1,3,15,20,28,31,35 — health policy, management, etc. e.g. 8,20,26,27,28,30,31 — conference proceedings e.g. 22,28,32 — reports e.g. 20,26,27,28,31.
5. **Case reports**	E. **Published reports** These cover 1–4, projects, special studies, etc.	
6. **'Data'** (statistics etc.)	F. **'Grey' literature** Theses, dissertations, reports, newsletters, circulars, etc.: may cover any of 1–6.	
	G. **Conference proceedings**	**Library catalogues** These cover E, G, monographs. Examples are 31,100 (Web).
	H. **Databases**, non-bibliographical This covers 6. Examples are 89,103,108, 109,110 (Web)	
	INTERNET World Wide Web sites provide increasing access to a whole range of primary and secondary resources in columns 2 and 3; examples are 76–140.	

Good information skills are the key to controlling this trade-off to advantage. We will focus on two essential types of information resource: the computer bibliographic database and the World Wide Web sites found on the Internet. Searchers often have difficulty finding information using these key resources, typically finding 'too little' or 'too much'.

Computer bibliographic databases

Computer bibliographic databases are our most important type of secondary resource. They give bibliographical details of material such as original studies, reviews and guidelines published in primary resources such as journals. As they increasingly become full-text databases delivering this original material from the search, they will become our most important primary resource. Issues of payment and copyright, rather than technology, delay this process. Databases contain huge amounts of data, with complex search software added by commercial vendors. Since no single database covers *all* journals in any field you often need to increase search sensitivity by searching several databases.

Many people find computer bibliographic databases such as MEDLINE, CINAHL or the Cochrane Library difficult to search. Others, more insidiously, do not find them as difficult as they ought to. There is evidence (McKibbon et al 1990, 1992, Shelstad & Clevenger 1994) from comparison of clinical searchers with information professionals that many searchers are not as skilled as they believe themselves to be, and often enter search strategies that are far too simple to retrieve the material they need. They blame databases for being unnecessarily difficult to search, believe they have not found the right 'keywords' (a much misused term) or feel that search software ought to think for them, that they lack 'computer' skills or that they simply do not have time for 'fancy searching'. While the mechanics of searching have become simpler with Windows-based systems (and improved Help facilities) it is good search skills and a basic understanding of databases that really make the difference.

The keys to effective searching are good strategy skills, transferable between databases and other resources. Once again, the structured clinical question provides an elegant framework for preparing a search strategy that we can use or develop for various databases, and even for Web search engines, many of which now mimic the advanced search features of databases. From the question we can find the best search terms and work out a strategy which we can broaden or narrow according to need and result. Search strategy development skills should take centre stage in the learning process, with computer operations merely the means to the end. This is the core of the teaching strategy we use in our Find the Evidence and Search Skills workshops at the Cairns Library in Oxford (Snowball 1997).

So let us prepare the HRT and osteoporosis question as a provisional search strategy:

Q. In post-menopausal women, does HRT prevent osteoporosis?

Table 3.2 Characteristics of patients (n = 4230) randomised to experimental or placebo treatment

Patient	Intervention	Outcome
postmenopausal	HRT	osteoporosis
post-menopausal	hormone replacement therapy	
post menopausal	hormone therapy/treatment	bone density
	oestrogen/s replacement/therapy	bone mineral density

After breaking the question into its main parts, we 'brainstorm' possible search terms for each part of the question. (A quick search, scanning titles and abstracts will always produce more terms: searching is an *iterative* or *cyclical* process.) Take care with less 'clinical' searches, which may have 'softer' terminology, that is, less term standardisation, vagueness, ambiguity or unclear overlap between related terms. Use more variant and related terms, and never rely only on the most obvious terms! We have all missed something important in a search, because we overlooked a relevant term.

Now we can use some basic search logic with the Boolean operators AND and OR, 'truncate' some word-endings and use 'wildcards' to construct our provisional search strategy. These are features common to many search systems, so we will have a seedbed of search terms and a basic strategy which we could use for searching other databases such as the Cochrane Library, EMBASE, MEDLINE or CINAHL, or even some Web search engines. MEDLINE is an excellent, general, health-care database, superb for developing search skills as it covers all health specialties, including nursing. (Brazier (1996) compares MEDLINE and CINAHL for nursing searches.) While the principles are similar, specific conventions or symbols may differ according to database, or to the search interfaces added to databases like MEDLINE by commercial vendors who provide CD-ROM or on-line access to the database. Checking the 'Help' facility first will always save you time and trouble!

We will use here the notation of SilverPlatter's MEDLINE (WinSpirs). The question mark is a 'wildcard' which stands in for one or no characters within words (useful for British/American English spellings such as h? emorrhage, and for inconsistently hyphenated terms). SilverPlatter's asterix (Ovid's dollar sign) is a 'truncation' or 'stemming' symbol, standing in for any number of characters (including none) at the end of a word –

essential if you don't want to miss the plural -s or -es of search terms or other useful word variants:

post?menopausal OR post menopausal
AND
hormone replacement therap* OR hormone therap* OR oestrogen* OR estrogen*
AND
Osteoporosis OR bone density OR bone mineral density

We link the most relevant terms with:

- OR: to retrieve records containing **any** of a set of terms (logical union of sets)
- AND: to retrieve records containing **all** of a set of terms, anywhere in the records (logical intersection of sets)
- NEAR: to retrieve records containing **both** terms, but in the same sentence of the record.

We can test out different combinations, amending our provisional strategy according to results, to *widen* or *narrow* the search as required: the very heart of searching. A skilled searcher will also continue to look for better search terms in retrieved records, to refine the search. So, on SilverPlatter we might first enter this strategy as:

#1 (oestrogen* or estrogen*) near (replacement or therap*) hormone*
#2 osteoporosis or bone density or bone mineral density
#3 #1 and #2

On MEDLINE and the Cochrane Library, this strategy produces about four times more references than a simple two-term search such as 'hormone replacement therapy and osteoporosis'. In MEDLINE (over 5 years), we retrieve 124 RCTs, 5 meta-analyses and 34 systematic reviews – as against 28 RCTs (thus missing a series of key trials), 3 meta-analyses and 12 systematic reviews. Think of the quality material – even one key review or meta-analysis – that we might miss with an overly simple search strategy! On the Cochrane Library, we find 40 trials with a simple two-term strategy, 160 using a MeSH term for HRT and including 'bone density', and 340 with a high-sensitivity strategy as above. So we are much less likely to miss trials, high-quality reviews and meta-analyses by starting with a *larger* number of retrievals. It is a common fault to narrow subject searching too much at the outset (often through lack of skill). We need to be able to construct a high-sensitivity search for finding the best evidence, especially if the literature on our topic is not large, and to be able to make it more specific when we need to do so – and vice versa.

The 'free-text' search ('Textword' on Ovid's Medline) or 'natural language' search is the basic search mode of most current search software. The secret is simply this: when you enter a term, e.g. 'osteoporosis', you will retrieve records *containing* that term, in, for example the title or abstract. This is not the same as retrieving records which are *about* osteoporosis! This is the key to understanding basic database searching. You get only what you put in: so with 'osteoporosis' you do not get 'bone density', or even 'osteoporotic'. It is a non-intelligent, character string search. Hence the need for covering all options with search term variants and truncation. Moreover, you will get records in which 'osteoporosis' is only mentioned in an abstract of an article which might have (for you) little to do with osteoporosis, or even in which it is mentioned to exclude it! Sensitivity can be too high – but you need high sensitivity if few studies have been published, as is so often the case.

So the next stage might be to increase search specificity. There are three ways to do this. First, you can refine your free-text search, by leaving out terms that increase sensitivity at the expense of specificity, retaining only the most relevant terms in the strategy. Second, you can try replacing any AND in your strategy which links terms you want more closely relating with NEAR, to retrieve terms which appear in the same sentence of titles or abstracts, and so are more likely to be semantically linked (e.g. nurs* near role*). Third, you can use the *Thesaurus* search, a higher level of search on many databases, which goes under various names ('Subject' on Ovid's Medline), and which remains unexplored by many searchers, who are, sadly, missing out on a powerful and sophisticated search tool.

The Thesaurus search matches your term to a standardised term used by trained indexers who have carefully read the original articles, and who use 'controlled terms' from a 'thesaurus' or term list to indicate significant subject content. So this search is the computer equivalent of looking up articles under a heading, (or 'about' a subject), as one does in the printed indexes, but with valuable additional features. On MEDLINE, we can look through the part of the record known as the MeSH (Medical Subject Headings) field – referred to as DE (Descriptor) on CINAHL, EMBASE and other databases – of relevant records we have already retrieved, to find useful index or MeSH terms. (Lowe & Barnett (1994) explain the use of MeSH in detail, including 'tree structures'.)

In our search, we quickly discover three MeSH terms which look useful, and so we amend our strategy for a Thesaurus search:

#1 Estrogen-Replacement-Therapy/all subheadings
#2 explode Osteoporosis/all subheadings ('explode' means 'include narrower terms': in this case Osteoporosis, Postmenopausal)
#3 Bone-Density/all subheadings
#4 #1 and (#2 or #3)

This will find only records indexed with these MeSH terms to indicate significant subject content, so producing a higher specificity search. Within the Thesaurus search, 'explosion' (usually a default option) increases sensitivity by searching narrower headings under broader ones. ('Exploding' Heart Diseases, for example, will search all MeSH headings for specific heart diseases, for extremely high sensitivity.)

Finally, 'subheadings' such as 'diagnosis', 'drug therapy', etc. can be added to qualify your headings, increasing specificity if selected singly, but increasing sensitivity if 'All Subheadings' are added. Some subheadings (therapy, diagnosis, etc.) relate directly to question types or study types, as do many main MeSH headings. Get to know them, or get a refresher session from your local health-care librarians!

The decision about how thorough your search should be is always *yours*. Clinicians may prefer the focus and speed of the Thesaurus, while researchers who want comprehensiveness will use complex free-text strategies, or combine both approaches, for maximum sensitivity. But a great deal also depends on the terminology of the topic and how it is used by authors, and the size and complexity of its literature. A higher sensitivity strategy is often needed, not to increase retrievals from, say, 50 to 400, but from 2 to 10! There may not be a useful Thesaurus term, especially for new developments, indexing quality varies, and not all databases have a Thesaurus-type option. (The Cochrane Library imports records with and without MeSH, so you must combine both approaches for each term when searching.) In general, you do need to be able to construct *both* high sensitivity and high specificity searches, using free text and Thesaurus, and to move skilfully between the extremes – if you do not want to miss that often elusive evidence!

Once you feel you have the best from your subject search – different strategies leading you back to the same material is one sign of this – then, on MEDLINE and CINAHL, you can use the Limit feature to focus on trials, RCTs, guidelines, systematic reviews and meta-analyses by 'publication type'.

You can also use 'search filters'. These are search strategies using research methodology terms in free text, Thesaurus or Limits (hence the alternative name 'methodologic filters') designed and tested to retrieve study types appropriate to diagnosis, prognosis, therapy, or aetiology/harm/risk. These are some of the very question types we started with – so here is a very strong link between question type and search strategy *within* key information resources.

Search filters are extremely useful when the literature on your topic is large. There are high sensitivity and high specificity versions, which can be saved to disk, and combined with your search. They are downloadable from some web sites (see (84) for links). On the Web MEDLINE, PubMED (140), they are usefully stored as Clinical Queries to add to searches. Those produced at McMaster University in Canada (McKibbon & Walker-Dilks

1993, 1994a, 1994b, McKibbon et al 1994, 1995, Walker-Dilks et al 1994) have been tested over a range of subjects, and published, most recently in a book by Anne McKibbon, containing her search filters for Medline, CINAHL, PsycINFO and EMBASE (McKibbon 1999). Any search may prove an exception to a general rule, so you may want to adapt a filter to increase sensitivity or specificity for your particular search.

For those who systematically review the literature, a comprehensive RCT strategy has been developed by the Cochrane Centre (available on the Cochrane Library – see Handbook), since RCTs have not always been clearly identified by authors or indexers, and many have only been traced by journal hand-searches. MEDLINE's 'publication type' randomised controlled trial only began to be used in 1991, since when many RCTs have been indexed retrospectively in MEDLINE (Dickerson et al 1995).

Using our developed osteoporosis strategy on MEDLINE yields some excellent trials and reviews, as well as original studies in which evidence remains buried. After MEDLINE, we might try EMBASE and CINAHL: a useful trio of databases for many health-care topics. Try BIOLOGICAL ABSTRACTS for life sciences research, ECONLIT for health economics studies, PSYCLIT for studies of psychological issues, BIOETHICSLINE for ethical and resources issues, and SOCIOFILE for health issues with a social emphasis, such as gerontology. Subject-specific databases (e.g. AIDSLINE, TOXLINE, AGEINFO) are also available. For clinical decisions, begin with the Cochrane Library, for high-quality reviews, and then try MEDLINE and other general or subject databases. Citation indexes such as Science Citation Index (42) trace the 'descendants' of an article by showing which authors have cited it. 'Grey' or unpublished literature is now so important that a major database, SIGLE (43), attempts to cope with the tip of this iceberg at least. Booth (1998) gives examples of following specific questions through various resources. These are key information skills that we *all* need to develop!

Coverage of even the larger databases can never be comprehensive: MEDLINE covers some 3900 published journals of a potentially relevant 20 000 and more! Specialised 'value-added' databases will continue to appear, such as the Cochrane Library which contains full-text systematic reviews, selective current awareness resources such as MD DIGESTS (34), INFORMED (73) and BEST EVIDENCE (7) allow clinicians to keep up with key papers relevant to clinical decision-making. There is an urgent need for clinical 'question-and-answer databases', containing 'frequently updated, evidence-based, peer-reviewed answers to specific common clinical questions' rather than full-text journal articles, according to Chambliss & Conley (1996: 144) who found that MEDLINE searches answered some three-quarters of their clinical questions in general practice, but that searching and appraising journal articles was 'time-consuming and expensive'. National databases of evidence-based guidelines would clearly be of enormous value for clinical practitioners. We also need to search across resources more easily: systems such as Doctors Desk (143) and TRIP (110) will develop further to allow access to a selection of high-quality resources at a sitting, to answer clinical questions more directly.

Database search software is becoming more sophisticated. The Boolean logic, term-retrieval and subject-heading model of current databases has long been contrasted with 'probabilistic' term searching (e.g. Hildreth 1989). Systems which match terms using 'fuzzy logic' will develop, but treat claims that they will 'think' for you with scepticism. Searching is really not an arcane process, and you can think through your search and find good search terms better than any software.

We will always need sound search skills. Most database searches need not take more than a few minutes. With a systematic approach, and a moderate investment of time to learn and practise, searching becomes fast and instinctive. It is a rewarding skill of enormous value, and can even be enjoyable. It depends less on being 'computer-literate' than on being able to find and test the best search terms, and broaden or narrow a search strategy at will. So, it is truly a *thinking* skill – not a mere computer skill!

World Wide Web sites

The growth of the Internet – that staggering global interconnection of computers in over 130 countries worldwide, of which the World Wide Web of information pages is a vital part – is fundamentally transforming the ways we disseminate and access information (see (108) on publishing). It offers access to personal, organisational, institutional and government web sites, prefaced by 'home-pages', which have links to further sites ad infinitum, and to downloadable software, searchable databases, learning packages, library catalogues, bibliographic databases, full-text 'electronic' journals, information gateways and 'virtual libraries' which organise information for easier access.

Once you have access to a computer with a graphical user interface such as Windows, a piece of software known as a web-'browser' which manages the operations of web-use, and web-connection via telephone line or network, three basic search operations are involved to find and visit web-pages:

1. clicking on 'hypertext links' (usually underlined words) on web-pages
2. typing in 'web-addresses' or Uniform Resource Locators (URLs)
3. using 'search engines' by entering search terms of your choice.

Some search engines, such as Alta-Vista (80), have Advanced Search features, using the ANDs, ORs, NEARs, and truncation of the databases, so allowing higher-specificity searches. Since there is generally no equivalent to the Thesaurus search (although OMNI has introduced MeSH indexing), you will need creative 'free-text' search skills, including trying different search terms, for effective searching. Searches on the Web can be slow and time-consuming because there is no 'telephone directory' of sites, and it can be difficult to get answers to specific questions. You may run into, as the saying goes, a lot of sewage before you hit clear surf! To cope with the chaos, more sophisticated 'meta-search' engines like Meta-Crawler (100), which use other search engines, are evolving, as are more focused 'medical' search engines like those on OMNI (105). Well-designed sites such as OncoLink (106) and other subject gateways offer clearly structured layout, browseable indexes – try those on Yahoo (113) – or subject menus and graphical site maps.

For our HRT and osteoporosis example, a quick OMNI search produces a dozen web sites with access to tutorials, organisations, bibliographies, reviews of epidemiological studies, clinical practice guidelines, links to more sites, and journals. (Journal Web sites may give more current information about the contents of specific journals than computer databases, because of the inevitable time delays of database entry.) For quality-of-life issues, try REGARD (41) and Glamm (91). Quality of information as evidence is extremely variable, but a web-search can supplement your database search in many ways. The two will merge seamlessly as more databases become web-accessible.

When you do find web pages, you face the crunch issues of authority and reliability of information. Anyone can set up a web site, and claim almost anything! Stick to the 'respectable' sites of academic, health service, professional and official organisations, and use specialist gateways such as OMNI which are likely to have vetted their information and links. Critically evaluate Web resources, carefully checking their support organisations or sponsors, and their update frequency, if you intend to use or cite information as evidence.

Having said this, the range of information is truly amazing, and growing fast, however long it takes to find it! The Select List of Information Resources (p. **34**) suggests gateways to many web sites. You might begin with Netting the Evidence (102), a treasure trove of evidence-based resources produced by Andrew Booth of ScHARR, who also produces an invaluable printed list of resources of all kinds (Booth 1997). Try an OMNI search to get started on a specific health topic, or on a general area such as 'guidelines' and browse OMNI Subject lists by specialty. Two books on health care and the Internet – Anthony (1996), good on technical aspects, and Kiley (1996), good on information resources, broader than its title suggests, and with its own updated web site, and the invaluable Health Information on the Internet (72) – will also help launch you on your fascinating journey into the infosphere!

REVIEWING THE SEARCH PROCESS

Finally, we must review the whole search process and evaluate each stage, revisiting each stage and repeating those we have doubts about. We may need to find and use further resources, and even reformulate our question, until we have the information which could be used as evidence to answer it – or until we are reasonably certain that it does not currently exist. Evidence-based practice, as we have seen, offers a model for these processes, and one in which doubts or knowledge gaps can be raised and dealt with objectively. But the certainty of a knowledge gap only increases with the thoroughness of our search for and within appropriate information resources, so we need at each stage to question resource appropriateness, coverage, currency, reliability and authority – as well as our own skills in finding and exploiting the resources effectively.

We may return to the problematic situation, but with a clearer understanding of the evidence currently available – the state of current 'knowledge'. A knowledge gap may usefully indicate that data which might reveal information which can be used as evidence might still have to be collected or produced. (Identifying 'questions of major importance to the NHS for which good research evidence is currently lacking' is of interest to the NHS R&D Health Technology Assessment Programme at Southampton University (122). However, we can only feel reasonably certain of search thoroughness if we are truly *able* to find information to use as evidence from a wide a range of resources appropriate to each question type and level, and to widen or narrow our search 'net' – both for and within resources – according to need, context and result. Unless we can do this, we cannot judge how comprehensive or exhaustive we actually are for a given search, nor accurately evaluate the search process and assess our own success in answering the question.

Evidence-based health-care practice and development are dependent on the ability to find and process appropriate kinds of information to use as evidence. The key information skills are:

- formulating a clear structured *question* to ground and guide the search
- identifying the *type* of question being asked
- recognising the type of *information* which could be used as evidence, from the strongest to the weakest, appropriate to each type of question
- recognising the type of *study* which would provide such information
- identifying (primary or secondary) *resources* which give the results of such studies
- exploiting modern information resources to get the best information by:

  1. developing high-sensitivity and high-specificity search *strategies* from the question

2. using the full capability of modern search *software*
- evaluating and refining the search stages until the question is answered or it is reasonably certain that the information does not exist.

Acknowledgements

I would like to acknowledge the great help given to me in writing this chapter by the following, who read drafts and made valuable comments: Andrew Booth of the Sheffield Centre for Health and Related Research (ScHARR), Reinhard Wentz of Charing Cross and Westminster Medical School Library, Robert Kiley of the Wellcome Trust Information Service, and two colleagues at the Cairns Library in Oxford: Anne Lusher, Enquiry Services Manager, and Stephen Clarke, IT Manager who has produced the Cairns Library Web site. Thanks are also due to Judy Palmer, Director of the Anglia and Oxford Health Care Libraries Unit, who got me involved in teaching in the early stages of the Oxford Cert. EBHC course. Comments on my drafts by other authors of this work, especially by the Editor, were also extremely stimulating. All remaining errors and unclarity are mine alone!

REFERENCES

Anthony D 1996 Health on the internet. Blackwell Science, Oxford

Booth A 1997 The ScHARR guide to evidence-based practice. (ScHARR Occasional Paper No. 97/2) ScHARR (School of Health and Related Research), University of Sheffield

Booth A 1998 Following the evidence trail: EBHC on the Internet. *He@lth* Information on the Internet 1(1) (URL: http://www.wellcome.ac.uk/healthinfo/)

Brazier H 1996 Selecting a database for literature searches in nursing: MEDLINE or CINAHL? Journal of Advanced Nursing 24: 868–875

Chambliss M L, Conley J 1996 Answering clinical questions. The Journal of Family Practice 43(2): 140–144

Dickerson K, Scherer R, Lefebvre C 1995 Identifying relevant studies for systematic reviews. In: Chalmers I, Altman D G (eds) Systematic reviews. BMJ Publishing Group, London, p17–36

Enkin M W, Jadad A R 1998 Using anecdotal information in evidence-based health care: Heresy or necessity? Annals of Oncology 9: 963–966

Goffman E 1961 Asylums: essays on the social situation of mental patients and other inmates. Anchor, New York

Hildreth C R 1989 Intelligent interfaces and retrieval methods for subject searching in bibliographic retrieval systems: prepared by Charles R. Hildreth for the Library of Congress. Advances in Library Information Technology, issue no. 2. Cataloging Distribution Service, Library of Congress, Washington DC

Kiley R 1996 Medical information on the Internet: a guide for health professionals. Churchill Livingstone, Edinburgh, (Web site: http://www.churchillmed.com/Books/MedInter/kiley.html)

Lowe H J, Barnett G O 1994 Understanding and using the Medical Subject Headings (MeSH) vocabulary to perform literature searches. Journal of the American Medical Association 271(14): 1103–1108

McKibbon K A et al 1990 How good are clinical MEDLINE searches? A comparative study of clinical end-user and librarian searches. Computers and Biomedical Research 23: 583–593

McKibbon K A et al 1992 A study to enhance clinical end-user MEDLINE search skills: design and baseline findings. In: Clayton P D (ed) Fifteenth annual symposium on computer applications in medical care: a conference of the American Medical Informatics Association, Washington DC, 1991. McGraw-Hill, New York

McKibbon K A, Walker-Dilks C J 1993 Panning for applied clinical research gold. Online July: 105–108

McKibbon K A, Walker-Dilks C J 1994a Beyond ACP Journal Club: How to harness MEDLINE for diagnostic problems. [Editorial]. ACP Journal Club Sept/Oct: A10–12 (Annals of Internal Medicine 121 Suppl 2)

McKibbon K A, Walker-Dilks C J 1994b Beyond ACP Journal Club: How to harness MEDLINE for therapy problems. [Editorial]. ACP Journal Club July/August: A10–12 (Annals of Internal Medicine 121 Suppl 1)

McKibbon K A et al 1995 Beyond ACP Journal Club: How to harness MEDLINE for prognosis problems. [Editorial]. ACP Journal Club Jul/Aug: A12–14

McKibbon K A 1999 PDQ Evidence-based principles and practice. BC Decker, Hamilton, Canada

Mulrow C 1987 The medical review article: state of the science. Annals of Internal Medicine 106: 485–488

Mulrow C D 1995 Rationale for systematic reviews. In: Chalmers I, Altman D G (eds) Systematic reviews. BMJ Publishing Group, London, p1

Oxman A D 1995 Checklists for review articles. In: Chalmers I, Altman D G (eds) Systematic reviews. BMJ Publishing Group, London: p75–85

Popay J, Williams G 1998 Qualitative research and evidence-based healthcare. Journal of the Royal Society of Medicine 91 (Suppl 35): 32–37

Richardson S W et al 1995 The well-built clinical question: a key to evidence-based decisions. [Editorial]. ACP Journal Club 123(3): A12–13

Richardson W S, Wilson M C 1997 On questions, background and foreground. Clinical Epidemiology and Biostatistics Nov: 6–7

Shelstad K R, Clevenger F W 1994 On-line strategies of third-year medical students: perception vs fact. Journal of Surgical Research 56: 338–344

Smith R 1991 Through the crystal ball darkly: medical journals and the future. In: Lock S (ed) The future of medical journals: in commemoration of 150 years of the British Medical Journal. BMJ Publishing Group, London p 187–210

Snowball R 1997 Using the clinical question to teach search strategy: fostering transferable conceptual skills in user education by active learning. Health Libraries Review 14(3): 167–172

Stern J M, Simes R J 1997 Publication bias: evidence of delayed publication in a cohort study of clinical research projects. British Medical Journal 315: 640–645

Walker-Dilks C J, McKibbon K A, Haynes R B 1994 Beyond ACP Journal Club: How to harness MEDLINE for etiology problems. [Editorial]. ACP Journal Club Nov/Dec: A10–11

Select List of Information Resources

DATABASES AND INDEXES, JOURNALS, BULLETINS, NEWSLETTERS AND WEB SITES

Databases (and Indexes)

(1) **ACP LIBRARY ON DISK** CD-ROM database, from American College of Physicians; contains BEST EVIDENCE (7), and ACP-approved Clinical Practice Guidelines, Common Diagnostic Tests, Common Screening Tests. Web site: http://www.acponline.org/

(2) **AGEINFO** CD-ROM database produced by Centre for Policy on Ageing: http://www.cpa.org.uk

(3) **AGENCY FOR HEALTH CARE POLICY & RESEARCH** Web-accessible database containing practice guidelines in full form, clinicians' guide and patients' guide versions: http://www.ahcpr.gov/

(4) **AIDSLINE** Database containing bibliographical citations to Government reports, meeting abstracts, books and theses on clinical and research aspects of AIDS, epidemiology, health policy, social issues, from 1980. On-line access from Knight-Ridder (144); CD-ROM from SilverPlatter (146) and Ovid (145). Web-access: US National Library of Medicine (101), HealthGate (94).

(5) **AMED** (Allied and Alternative Medicine Database) British Library Database, CD-ROM (SilverPlatter), disk and printed versions. Bibliographical citations from over 400 journals covering wide range of alternative and complementary health practice.

(6) **ASSIA** (Applied Social Sciences Index & Abstracts) CD-ROM database from Bowker-Saur, (on-line from Knight-Ridder), containing bibliographical citations from 500+ English-language journals from 16 countries on nursing, social work, sociology, social and economic aspects of health care, communication, education, ethnic studies, psychology etc., from 1987. Details on Web site: http://www.bowker-saur.co.uk/service/cdrom/assia/htm

(7) **BEST EVIDENCE** Full-text database, disk or CD-ROM, produced by American College of Physicians and British Medical Journal Publishing, available from BMA. Contains all articles from two 'secondary' review journals – ACP Journal Club (from January 1991) and Evidence-Based Medicine (from 1995) – over wide range of medical specialties, with abstracts and comments by clinical experts, editorials on critical appraisal and clinical application, glossary of statistical terms with examples.

(8) **BIOETHICSLINE** CD-ROM (SilverPlatter, Ovid), online (Ovid, Knight-Ridder) and Web-accessible database from US National Library of Medicine and Kennedy Institute of Ethics, Georgetown University. Contains bibliographical citations to articles on ethical issues, public policy and resource allocation in medicine, health care and biomedical research, including new reproductive technologies, genetic engineering, abortion, behaviour control, mental health therapies, human experimentation. Over 44 000 records, 1973 onwards, from range of sources, including 40 journals not indexed on Medline. Free Web-access on HealthGate (94): http://www.healthgate.co.uk/medline/search-adv.shtml

(9) **BIOLOGICAL ABSTRACTS** Huge database of references and abstracts of articles from over 6000 journals, 1985 onwards, all aspects of life sciences. BIOSIS Previews and BIOSIS GenRef for genetics also available. CD-ROM (SilverPlatter); on-line access (Knight-Ridder). Covers biotechnology, genetics, immunology, neuroscience, pharmacology, toxicology, microbiology, clinical and experimental medicine, biochemistry, biophysics, environmental studies, etc.

(10) **BRITISH NURSING INDEX** Printed index, CD-ROM and Web-accessible database covering some 220 English-language journals in nursing, midwifery and community health care received at the libraries of Bournemouth University, Royal College of Nursing Library and health-care libraries in Salisbury and Dorset, indexed within 6 weeks of publication. Index from BNI Publications, University of Bournemouth. CD-ROM and Web version produced by BNI Publications and Optology Ltd, by subscription: http://www.optology.com

(11) **CAB HEALTH** CD-ROM (SilverPlatter) and on-line (Knight-Ridder) database of bibliographical citations from 11 000+ journals from 130 countries, 1973 onwards, on communicable diseases and disease control, tropical and parasitic diseases, nutrition, medicinal and poisonous plants, environmental and public health.

(12) **CENTRE FOR RESEARCH IN ETHNIC RELATIONS DATABASE** Web-accessible ethnic health database compiled by Warwick University Clinical Sciences Library: http://www.warwick.ac.uk/fac/soc/CRER RC/search.html

(13) **CENTRE FOR REVIEWS AND DISSEMINATION (CRD) DATABASES** The UK National Health Service Centre for Reviews and Dissemination (CRD), University of York, produces and disseminates reviews on effectiveness and cost-effectiveness of specific health-care interventions, health-care delivery and health-care technology from high-quality health research for decision-makers and health consumers. CRD databases, Web-accessible or dial-up: DARE (also on Cochrane Library): high-quality systematic reviews,

summaries of authors' conclusions and comments on practice implications; NEED: database of economic evaluations. CRD Web site: http://www.york.ac.uk/inst/crdwelcome.htm

(14) CHILDDATA CD-ROM database (quarterly updates, by subscription) with details of organisations, news, conferences, index to wide range of published information from National Children's Bureau, who also produce ChildData Abstracts, a monthly printed listing of publications and research in child welfare topics: http://www.ncb.org.uk

(15) CINAHL (Cumulative Index to Nursing & Allied Health Literature) Key CD-ROM (SilverPlatter, Ovid) and on-line (Knight-Ridder) database. Bibliographical citations (with abstracts and reference lists) from nursing and allied health-care journals, conference proceedings, standards of professional practice, guidelines (full-text), nursing dissertations, from 1982.

(16) COCHRANE DATABASE OF SYSTEMATIC REVIEWS Available on Cochrane Library (17). Separately available on Web by subscription: Synapse Publishing: http://www.wepublish.com/jmb/default.htm

(17) COCHRANE LIBRARY Databases of the international Cochrane Collaboration, computer disk or CD-ROM (from British Medical Journal Publishing Group, search interface from Update Software, Oxford). Suite of 4 databases:

1. Cochrane Database of Systematic Reviews (CDSR): full-text systematic reviews of effects of health-care interventions in pregnancy and childbirth, stroke, schizophrenia, and increasing range of specialties;
2. York Database of Abstracts & Reviews of Effectiveness (DARE): structured abstracts of high quality published systematic reviews;
3. Cochrane Controlled Trials Register (CCTR): bibliographies of 150 000 controlled trials, many not listed in major biomedical databases (see also Medical Editors' Trials Amnesty for some 150 unpublished trials);
4. Cochrane Review Methodology Database (CRMD): bibliography of articles on research methodology and preparing systematic reviews.

Also includes Cochrane Collaboration Handbook and ScHARR Netting the Evidence Guide to EBP Sources on the Internet (102 below). Web site: http://www.cochrane.co.uk

(18) CURRENT CONTENTS Set of databases on computer disk (ISI), on-line access (Knight-Ridder, Ovid), CD-ROM (SilverPlatter, Ovid) and hard-copy journal, produced by ISI (Institute for Scientific Information). Wide subject range: life sciences, clinical medicine, etc. Contains journal contents pages, updated monthly (disks), weekly (hard-copy version), for references (no abstracts) to very recently published material, often prior to appearance in databases. Current ISI search software allows searching of only one issue at a time on disk, but ISI are developing new product: 'Web of Science'.

(19) DATABASE OF ABSTRACTS & REVIEWS OF EFFECTIVENESS (DARE) See Cochrane Library (17), and Centre for Reviews and Dissemination Databases (13).

(20) DoH-DATA On-line database of UK Department of Health. Huge number of bibliographic citations on all aspects of health care, management, policy, national guidelines, etc. On-line (Knight-Ridder); part of HMIC Database (31).

(21) DISSERTATION ABSTRACTS Database of over 1.2 million citations with abstracts to doctoral theses, masters' theses, and other dissertations from North American, Canadian and international educational institutions, all disciplines. On-line (Knight-Ridder) and CD-ROM (SilverPlatter, Ovid) access.

(22) ECONLIT Database from American Economic Association containing citations from 400+ economics and related journals, books, book reviews, conference proceedings and working papers, from 1969. Web-accessible, with CD-ROM (SilverPlatter, Ovid) and on-line access (Ovid, Knight-Ridder).

(23) EMBASE Key general biomedical and pharmacological database produced by Elsevier Science, containing citations and abstracts from 3500 journals from 70 countries, 1980 onwards; strong coverage of European journals. Available on-line (Knight-Ridder, Ovid) and CD-ROM (SilverPlatter, Ovid); subsets for main medical specialties, and Embase Alert (bi-weekly updates of most recent items) also offered.

(24) ERIC Database of educational literature, sponsored by US Department of Education. Contains Resources in Education (RIE), Current Index to Journals in Education (CIJE) covering published literature from over 775 journals, 1966 onwards, and ERIC Digests for overviews of educational topics with references. Available on-line BIDS (82), (Ovid, Knight-Ridder, who also offer British Education Index) and CD-ROM (SilverPlatter, Ovid).

(25) EXTRAMED Full-text database of 200+ biomedical journals, mainly from developing countries, result of WHO initiative. Covers tropical diseases, traditional medicine, bio-diversity, communicable diseases, health development studies, 1993 onwards. On-line (Knight-Ridder) and CD-ROM access (Microinfo Ltd).

(26) HEALTH SERVICE ABSTRACTS Monthly printed abstracting bulletin; bibliographical details and summaries of books, reports, journal articles and other publications on the non-clinical aspects of health services, with main emphasis on UK. Lists Department of Health publications, including circulars and statistical bulletins: details on Web site: http://www.open/gov.uk/doh/dhhome.htm

(27) HEALTH-CD Full-text database (CD-ROM from SilverPlatter) produced by UK Stationery Office and Department of Health; unique source of legislation, guidance notes, newsletters, reports on UK health management and health care.

(28) HEALTHSTAR Web-accessible (Healthgate (94), National Library of Medicine (101), CD-ROM (SilverPlatter, Ovid), and on-line (Knight-Ridder) database from National Library of Medicine, Bethesda, USA. (Formerly HealthPlan: from 1996 includes HEALTH and HSTAR databases.) Non-clinical aspects of health-care policy, planning, administration, delivery, and economics, health services research, clinical practice guidelines, quality assurance, health care technology assessment, etc. from journals, books, technical and official reports, conference papers, newspaper articles, from 1975 or most recent 10 years.

(29) HEED (HEALTH ECONOMIC EVALUATIONS DATABASE) CD-ROM database from Office of Health Economics (UK) and International Federation of Pharmaceutical Manufacturers Associations (OHE/IFPMA). Contains 6000+ bibliographical references, 2000+ reviewed articles, with analysis of key articles, on health economics, including cost-effectiveness studies and other forms of economic evaluation. Web site: http://www.abpi.org.uk/ohe.htm

(30) HELMIS On-line database of Nuffield Institute for Health: covers UK health-care management and quality issues. Available by subscription: Nuffield Institute for Health, 71–75 Clarendon Road, Leeds LS2 9PL, and included in HMIC Database (31). Web site: http://www.leeds.ac.uk/nuffield/home.html

(31) HMIC (Health Management Information Consortium) Set of three databases: DoH Data (from UK Department of Health: 20), HELMIS (from Nuffield Institute for Health: 31) and King's Fund Library catalogue. References from journals, books, reports, official publications, and 'grey' literature, covering health service policy, management, organisation, finance, quality of care etc. in primary, public and community care, from 1983. CD-ROM and Web access (SilverPlatter).

(32) INDEX TO SCIENTIFIC & TECHNICAL PROCEEDINGS Bibliographical references to papers from 4000+ conferences annually: wide range of science-related subjects, 1982 onwards, via BIDS (82), and as a printed index.

(33) INDEX TO THESES OF GREAT BRITAIN & IRELAND Database of references (some abstracts) to theses and dissertations submitted to UK and Irish universities and colleges. Covers contents of printed Index to Theses (Portland Press) from 1970, vol. 21. No updated CD-ROM. Web-access via personal or institutional subscription: http://www.theses.com/

(34) MD DIGESTS Web-accessible 'database' containing clinically focused summaries of selected articles from 'the top five medical' journals, with MEDLINE abstracts, updated weekly; offers Related Links to Web sites relevant to topic, Related Literature Search of topic on selected databases, plus citations and abstracts of author's previously published articles. Web site: http://php2.silverplatter.com/digintro.htm

(35) MEDLINE Database version of printed indexes Index Medicus and International Nursing Index, produced by US National Library of Medicine. Key general health database, covering clinical medicine, health care, nursing and midwifery, of bibliographical citations (80% with abstracts) from 3900 journals worldwide, 1966 onwards. Available on CD-ROM (SilverPlatter, Ovid), on-line access (e.g. Knight-Ridder), and Web-access (e.g. 93, 94, 100, 105, 136 below) to part or whole of database, with variable search facilities.

(36) META-REGISTER OF CONTROLLED TRIALS (mRCT) Web-accessible database of ongoing controlled trials in progress from a range of trials registers, produced by Current Controlled Trials Ltd, London. Search or browse the 'meta-register': http://www.controlled-trials.com/home.htm

(37) NHS ECONOMIC EVALUATION DATABASE (NEED) Web-accessible database (previously Department of Health Register of Cost-effectiveness Studies). Contains some 1000+ published economic evaluations and studies of health-care interventions, identified and reviewed by health economists and information specialists, with structured summaries, quality assessment, and details of practical implications. Access via CRD Databases on NHS Centre for Reviews & Dissemination Web site: http://www.york.ac.uk/inst/crd/

(38) NHS RESEARCH REGISTER Suite of databases on CD-ROM of current UK NHS-funded research. Free from regional NHS R&D Directorates, under NHS R&D Programme's Information Systems Strategy. Contains National Research Register Projects Database, MRC Clinical Trials Directory, Register of Registers, Register of Reviews in Progress, and Health Research at York Database. Cochrane-style search interface from Update Software. Prototype August 1997 quarterly from 1999. Networkable without licence.

(39) PSYCLIT Database derived from American Psychological Association's comprehensive information resource PsycINFO. (Printed index: Psychological Abstracts.) References and abstracts of articles from 1300 journals from 50 countries, and from published books, on psychology and related disciplines, 1974 onwards, updated quarterly. ClinPSYC: subset of PsycLIT, covering medical and psychological disorders and treatment. PsycINFO available on-line (Knight-Ridder, Ovid), PsycLIT on CD-ROM (SilverPlatter, Ovid). APA products available by subscription from APA: Web site: http://www.apa.org/

(40) QUALITY OF LIFE ASSESSMENT IN MEDICINE CD-ROM database produced by Glamm Interactive, Italy: 9000 references from last 20 years, and 100+ evaluation instruments. (Subscription approx. US$200.) Useful Web site with links to related sites: http://www.glamm.com/ql/

(41) REGARD Web-accessible database developed at University of Bristol, funded by Economic and Social Research Council (ESRC); contains details of ESRC-funded research awards and projects in wide range of social sciences and related research, and resultant publications; publicly accessible free of charge: http://www.regard.ac.uk/

(42) SCIENCE CITATION INDEX Citation Indexes allow you to find papers cited by other authors, and allow general searching. Science Citation Index, Social Sciences Citation Index, and Arts and Humanities Citation Index appear in printed form; on-line access via BIDS (82), and as SciSearch and Social SciSearch (both with added records from Current Contents) from Knight-Ridder Information.

(43) SIGLE (System for Information on Grey Literature in Europe) Database (CD-ROM from SilverPlatter) produced by EAGLE (European Association for Grey Literature Exploitation), a consortium of major European libraries, of reports, dissertations and other 'grey' literature not widely published, and difficult to identify and obtain. Wide subject coverage. All entries have availability details, including British Library shelfmarks.

SOCIAL SCIENCE CITATION INDEX See (42) above.

(44) SOCIOFILE Database from Sociological Abstracts Inc. Citations with abstracts from 2300 journals published since 1974, dissertations from 1986, association papers, books, films and software relevant to theoretical and applied sociology, social policy, social aspects of health. CD-ROM (SilverPlatter, Ovid). Sociological abstracts also available on-line (Knight-Ridder, Ovid).

(45) TOXLINE: Database of 2 million bibliographical records, 1965 on, from National Library of Medicine and other sources. Covers toxicological effects of drugs, chemicals, and physical agents; adverse drug reactions, carcinogenesis, environmental pollution, food contamination, water treatment, pesticides, herbicides, risk assessment, etc. CD-ROM (SilverPlatter), on-line (Knight-Ridder).

Journals

A selection of recent journals with a strong 'evidence-based' or review interest. Many have useful Web sites!

(46) ACP JOURNAL CLUB (ISSN 0003-4819) Secondary bi-monthly journal from American College of Physicians, containing summaries of significant articles 'that warrant immediate attention by physicians attempting to keep pace with important advances in treatment, prevention, diagnosis, cause, prognosis and economics of the disorders managed by internists' from 50 major medical journals, with expert commentary on practice perspectives and editorials on evidence-based practice issues (see Best Evidence). Web site: http://www.acponline.org/journals/acpic/jcmenu.htm

(47) CLINICAL EFFECTIVENESS IN NURSING (ISSN 1361-9004) Monthly primary journal published by Churchill Livingstone. Peer-reviewed articles with commentaries on clinical interventions and outcomes in all specialties.

(48) CLINICAL PERFORMANCE AND QUALITY HEALTHCARE Official quarterly journal of Society for Healthcare Epidemiology of America. Peer-reviewed articles combining quality improvement strategies and clinical research. Covers quality of health care, EBHC, outcomes research, decision analysis, application of practice guidelines and clinical pathways, appropriateness of care.

(49) CONTROLLED CLINICAL TRIALS (incorporating CLINICAL TRIALS & METAANALYSIS) (ISSN 0197-2456) Official monthly journal of the Society for Clinical Trials, published by Elsevier Science; articles on design, methods, operational aspects of controlled clinical trials and follow-up studies, and associated operational, methodological, legal and ethical problems and solutions. Web site: http://www.elsevier.nl:80/inca/publications/store/5/0/5/7/5/8/

CURRENT CONTENTS Hard-copy secondary journal: see (18) above.

(50) DISEASE MANAGEMENT AND HEALTH OUTCOMES Monthly journal published by Adis International; forum for collating, evaluating and disseminating practical knowledge on disease management based on best evidence. Includes research into outcomes measurement, and information on management programmes. Web site: http://www.adis.com.uk

(51) EVIDENCE-BASED CARDIOVASCULAR MEDICINE (ISSN 1361-2611) Quarterly secondary journal published by Churchill Livingstone. Summaries of key, high-quality articles with commentaries on cardiovascular topics, and educational articles on evidence-based practice.

(52) EVIDENCE-BASED HEALTH POLICY AND MANAGEMENT (ISSN 1363-4038) Quarterly secondary journal published by Churchill Livingstone. Summaries of key articles on health policy and management, and educational articles on evidence-based practice, to provide managers with best available evidence on financing, organisation, delivery of health care. Web site: http://www.ihs.ox.ac.uk/jebhpm/

(53) EVIDENCE-BASED MEDICINE (ISSN 1356-5524) Bi-monthly secondary journal published by BMJ Publishing Group and American College of Physicians. Summaries of key original and review articles from the biomedical literature, with commentaries by clinical experts, alerting clinicians to important advances over wide range of medical specialties. (See Best Evidence (7) above.) Web site: http://www.bmjpg.com/data/ebm.htm

(54) EVIDENCE-BASED MENTAL HEALTH Quarterly secondary journal in mental health issues from Centre for Evidence-Based Mental Health, Oxford and BMJ Publishing Group, for full range of clinicians, therapists, managers and policy makers. Some articles full text on Web site (134) below.

(55) EVIDENCE-BASED NURSING (ISSN 1367-6539) Quarterly secondary journal, published by RCN Publishing Company and BMJ Publishing Group, from January 1998. Identifies and appraises high quality, clinical research articles published in primary journals, with critical abstracts, and commentaries by practising nurses.
EVIDENCE-BASED PURCHASING See (71) below.
(56) GENERAL PRACTICE ON-LINE The International Journal of General Practice (ISSN: 1359-7631) One of a range of free registration, peer-reviewed Web journals from Priory Lodge Education:
http://www.priory.com/gp.htm
(57) JOURNAL OF CLINICAL EFFECTIVENESS (ISSN 1361-5874) Quarterly multidisciplinary primary journal (previously Medical Audit News), from Churchill Livingstone. Articles on evidence and practice, clinical effectiveness, guidelines and clinical audit, over range of disciplines.
(58) JOURNAL OF CLINICAL EPIDEMIOLOGY (ISSN 0895-4356) Monthly primary journal from Elsevier Science. Authoritative studies relating to clinical medicine, epidemiology, biostatistics and pharmacoepidemiology, including Pharmacoepidemiology Reports for rapid publication of articles on clinical epidemiologic investigations of pharmaceutical agents. Web site:
http://www.elsevier.nl:80/inca/publications/store/5/2/5/4/7/2/
(59) JOURNAL OF EVALUATION IN CLINICAL PRACTICE (ISSN 1365-2753) Monthly primary journal from Blackwell Science. Articles promoting critical enquiry into, and evaluation of, clinical practice in medicine, nursing and other health professions. Web site:
http://www.blacksci.co.uk/products/journals/jecp.htm
(60) THE JOURNAL OF FAMILY PRACTICE Monthly journal, Web-accessible and hard-copy forms. Reviews and critically appraises key articles, selected for potential to change practice, from 80 primary care journals. Recommendations for clinical practice: POEMs (Patient-Oriented Evidence that Matters). Web site provides e-mail discussion of issues raised by articles, EBP Newsletter, good primary care links:
http://jfp.msu.edu/
(61) JOURNAL OF HEALTH SERVICES RESEARCH AND POLICY (ISSN 1355-8196) Quarterly journal published by Churchill Livingstone. Original articles on health services research and policy for practitioners, managers, policy-makers.
(62) JOURNAL OF QUALITY IN CLINICAL PRACTICE (ISSN 1320-5455) Quarterly journal published by Blackwell Science. Original articles on issues and developments in health-care quality, health policies, and health-care delivery, with abstracts, news and comments on clinical review meetings. Web site:
http://www.blacksci.co.uk/products/journals/xjqcp.htm
(63) NT RESEARCH (ISSN 1361-4096) Sister journal to Nursing Times, published bi-monthly by Macmillan Magazines, from 1996. Original clinical research papers on wide range of nursing and related areas, with review articles and critical commentary by academic peers.
(64) ONLINE JOURNAL OF CURRENT CLINICAL TRIALS On-line journal published by Chapman & Hall, containing peer-reviewed primary research studies, reviews, meta-analyses, methodological papers, editorials, information on trials in medicine and allied health. Details on Web site:
http://www.coalliance.org/unitrec/ej000225.html

Bulletins and Newsletters

(65) BANDOLIER Monthly bulletin published by Oxford and Anglia NHS Region, containing summaries and bullet points (hence title!) on drug and treatment interventions and EBHC matters of interest, for purchasers. Web-version:
http://www.jr2.ox.ac.uk/Bandolier
(66) CLINICAL EPIDEMIOLOGY NEWSLETTER Continues as EVIDENCE-BASED HEALTHCARE NEWSLETTER (70).
(67) COCHRANE COLLABORATION NEWSLETTERS Range of newsletters from Cochrane Centres, Collaborative Review Groups, Methods Working Groups, and others:
http://www.update-software.com/ccweb/cochrane/newslet.htm

(68) **EFFECTIVE HEALTH CARE BULLETIN** (ISSN 0965–0288) Bulletin published eight times annually by CT Healthcare, addressing effectiveness of interventions on a major health-care topic, with systematic reviews. Also full-text on NHS Centre for Reviews and Dissemination Web site:
http://www.york.ac.uk/inst/crd/dissem.htm

(69) **EFFECTIVENESS MATTERS** Occasional peer-reviewed bulletins published by NHS Centre for Reviews and Dissemination, University of York (103) and subject experts.

(70) **EVIDENCE-BASED HEALTHCARE NEWSLETTER** (Previously CLINICAL EPIDEMIOLOGY NEWSLETTER) Published by Department of Clinical Epidemiology and Biostatistics, McMaster University, covers range of issues in teaching and practising evidence-based healthcare. Web site:
http://hiru.mcmaster.ca/ceb/

(71) **EVIDENCE-BASED PURCHASING** Bi-monthly newsletter from NHS Executive, South and West Research and Development Directorate: digest of selected material commissioned or from journals about effective care, to support commissioning role. Available from Information and Communications Co-ordinator, Research and Development Directorate, Canynge Hall, Whiteladies Road, Bristol. Text and subject index on Web site:
http://cochrane.epi.bris.ac.uk/rd/publicat/ebpurch/index.htm

(72) **HE@LTH INFORMATION ON THE INTERNET** Published by Wellcome Trust and Royal Society of Medicine, from February 1998. Bookmarks: links, new sites, original articles on health care and the Internet, discussion lists; details:
http://www.wellcome.ac.uk/healthinfo

(73) **INFORMED** (ISSN 1201-2475) Quarterly newsletter produced by Institute of Clinical Evaluative Sciences (ICES), Toronto, Canada. Aims to 'put health services information and clinical research together in a clear and concise format' for practising physicians, on range of medical topics. Hard-copy version Can$40 annually outside Canada; Web-accessible from:
http://www.ices.on.ca/

(74) **OUTCOMES BRIEFING** Bi-annual publication from UK Clearing House on Health Outcomes, Nuffield Institute for Health, University of Leeds, 71–75 Clarendon Road, Leeds LS2 9PL. Current awareness, conference report, workshops, report on work of Clearing House, articles and debate on outcomes issues. Web site:
http://www.leeds.ac.uk/nuffield/infoservices/UKCH/publi.html

(75) **PROMOTING ACTION ON CLINICAL EFFECTIVENESS (PACE)** 3-year programme funded by NHS executive at King's Fund Development Centre, London, examining change in clinical behaviour. Free quarterly progress Bulletins; interim report 'Turning evidence into everyday practice' outlines findings from 1st year of 16 UK development sites, each working on treatment of specific conditions: from King's Fund bookshop.

Internet Discussion Lists/Support Groups:

Join a discussion list to contact experts, debate current issues, exchange information or simply 'lurk'. Andrew Booth of ScHARR (see 102) has a directory of EBH-related lists at:
http://www.shef.ac.uk/~scharr/ir/email.html See also (60), (72), (86), (104).

(76) **Mailbase** (e-mail: mailbase@mailbase.ac.uk; Web site: http://www.mailbase.ac.uk/) run lists such as: evidence-based-health, health-services-research, nurse-decision, GP-UK and many others.

(77) **Doctors.Net** Forum, search engine, library, news, jobs, database and journals access for GMC members:
http://www.doctors.net.uk/

(78) **Evidence-Based Family Planning Discussion List**
http://www.nthames-health.tpmde.ac.uk/ebfp/

(79) **New Interactive Forum for all UK health professionals** Web discussion boards, chat rooms and more:
http://anexa.paralogic.com/ukhealthcentre/index.html

Web sites

See also Web-addresses in sections above. Inclusion of any web site is *not* a guarantee of reliability or authority!

'Gateways' and Search Engines

(80) Alta-Vista General search engine, with Advanced Search feature:
http://altavista.com/

(81) The Best Medical Sites on the Web Reviewed list of sites produced by editors at Priory Lodge Education:
http://www.priory.com/other.htm

(82) BIDS Bath Information and Data Services: Journals on-line (full-text electronic journals) and bibliographic databases in medicine, social sciences etc., mainly subscription-based, for academic users:
http://www.bids.ac.uk

BioMedNet See (138) below.

(83) British Healthcare Internet Association
http://bhia.org/

(84) Cairns Library, Oxford Health Links to sites in this list and others, search engines, electronic journals, search filters, guides:
http://www.medicine.ox.ac.uk/cairns

(85) CASP Critical Appraisal Skills for Purchasers: premier site for critical appraisal issues, materials, workshops, links:
http://www.ihs.ac.uk/casp/

(86) Centre for Psychotherapeutic Studies Links to 15 000 resources, distance education, mental health bookshop, journals search, on-line dictionary of mental health (links to 860 psychology, psychiatry, neuroscience, social science journals, and mental health texts), mental health search engine, discussion groups:
http://www.shef.ac.uk/~psyc/

(87) Children with Diabetes Model site layout: latest research, news, searches:
http://www.castleweb.com/diabetes/

(88) CliniWeb Index and table of contents to clinical information on the Web, search engine or browse using MeSH; links to Medline:
http://www.ohsu.edu/cliniweb

(89) Department of Health (UK) Publications, events, press releases, statistics sources, search engine:
http://www.open.gov.uk/doh/dhhome.htm

(90) Family PlanNet Evidence-based resources: links, discussion list:
http://www.nthames-health.tpmde.ac.uk/Family PlanNet/

(91) Glamm Interactive Producers of database Quality of Life Assessment in Medicine, see (40): Internet resources links to related sites, directories, journals, assessment instruments, organisations, research groups and more:
http://www.glamm.com/ql/url.htm

(92) Health Centre 'Clinic' for links to patient/consumer-related sites; 'Staff Room' for health-care professional links:
http://www.healthcentre.org.uk

(93) Health Communication Network Access to Medline, Cochrane (subscription), library of information: health books, education packages, on-line journals, world conference calendar, search engines:
http://www.hen.net.au

(94) Healthgate Wide range of links, subject index, access to databases: Medline, AidsLine, Bioethicsline, CancerLit, HealthStar:
http://www.healthgate.com/HealthGate/home.html

He@lth Information on the Internet See 72.

(95) Internet Biomedical News News about latest Internet biomedical information resources, monthly, by subscription:
http://www.ic.uk.com/lifebase/ibn.htm

(96) Internet Resources Newsletter Free Web resource for general users: news, sites, reviews, etc. Latest issue:
http://www.hw.ac.uk/libWWW/irn/irn39/irn39.html
(97) Journal of Family Practice See 60: excellent primary care links and more:
http://jfp.msu.edu/
(98) Medical World Search Search 100 000 full-text Web pages from thousands of high-quality medical sites:
http://www.mwsearch.com
(99) Medicine and the Internet On-line updates of Oxford University Press book 'Medicine and the Internet' by McKenzie (1997): search features, links, Internet technical information:
http://wwwl.oup.co.uk/scimed/medint/
(100) MetaCrawler One of a new generation of meta-search engines:
http://www.metacrawler.com/
(101) National Library of Medicine, Bethesda, USA Medline, book catalogues, databases and more:
http://www.nlm.nih.gov/
(102) Netting the Evidence A goldmine from Andrew Booth, School of Health and Related Research (ScHARR), University of Sheffield:
http://www.shef.ac.uk/uni/academic/R-Z/scharr/ir/netting.html
(Included on Cochrane Library, See 17). See also ScHARR Trawling the Net:
http://www.shef.ac.uk/~scharr/ir/trawling.html and ScHARR-Lock's Guide to the Evidence:
http://www.shef.ac.uk/uni/academic/R-Z/scharr/ir/scebm.html
(103) NHS Centre for Reviews and Dissemination CRD Databases, publications, bibliography, links:
http://www.york.ac.uk/inst/crd/
(104) Nursing & Health Care Resources on the Net Over 1000 Web sites, mailing lists and newsgroups for nurses and all health care professionals, strong UK content:
http://www.shef.ac.uk/~nhcon
(105) OMNI Major 'gateway,' with specialist search engines for Internet resources in medicine, bio-sciences, allied health, health management etc.: claims comprehensive coverage of reliable UK and worldwide health resources. Browse subject lists for current awareness; regular Newsletter:
http://omni.ac.uk/
(106) OncoLink A 'multimedia oncology information resource'; plethora of links, disease and specialty-oriented menus, FAQs, health consumer information, journals, search engine; award-winning example of Web site information sign-posting and layout; splendid resource for oncology-related searching:
http://cancer.med.upenn.edu/
(107) OXAMWEB Oxford and Anglia Mental Health Web: Internet library of evidence-based mental health information: EB logo to mark sites and documents meeting quality evidence criteria:
http://strauss.ihs.ox.ac.uk/oxamweb.html
(108) Scholarly Electronic Publishing Bibliography Articles on publishing and the Internet:
http://info.lib.uh.edu/sepb/sepb.html
(109) SOSIG (Social Science Information Gateway) On-line catalogue: search and browse access to thousands of quality Internet resources, including statistics sources, over wide range of social science and related areas:
http://sosig.ac.uk
(110) TRIP (Turning Resource into Practice) Database of hypertext links compiled from 18 key, evidence-based practice sources – Bandolier, Cochrane Database of Systematic Reviews, Journal of Family Practice, etc. Title search only. On-line newsletter; 1150+ links:
http://www.gwent.nhs.gov.uk/trip/
(111) User Guides to the Medical Literature Full list of EBHC guides published in JAMA 1993–7: links to full-text versions at McMaster University, Canada:
http://www.shef.ac.uk/~scharr/ir/userg.html
(112) World Health Organization WHO Reports, statistics, library search, information sources, links, search engine:
http://www.who.org/

(113) Yahoo General search engine, browseable subject links:
http://www.yahoo.com/

Guidelines

See also Royal Colleges Web sites for specific subject guidelines.

(114) Agency for Health Care Policy & Research (AHCPR) See (3) above:
http://www.ahcpr.gov/
(115) Canadian Co-ordinating Office for Health Technology Assessment 'Guidelines for Economic Evaluation of Pharmaceuticals: Canada':
http://www.ccohta.ca.
(116) Canadian Medical Association Clinical Practice Guidelines Database and Canadian Task Force on Preventive Health Care
http://www.cma.ca/cpgs/
(117) CancerNet Physician Data Query
http://wwwicic.nci.nih.gov/
(118) Centres for Disease Control and Prevention (CDC) Guidelines Database Up-to-date comprehensive repository of all official guidelines and recommendations published by US Centres for Disease Control and Prevention:
http://aepo-xdv-www.epo.cdc.gov/wonder/prevguid/prevguid.htm
(119) Guideline Developing database of guidelines based at Institute of Health Sciences Library, Oxford, critically appraised using appraisal instrument developed by Health Care Evaluation Unit, St George's Hospital Medical School (120):
http://www.ihs.ox.ac.uk/guidelines/index.html
(120) Health Care Evaluation Unit, Department of Public Health Sciences, St George's Hospital Medical School Appraisal Instrument for Clinical Guidelines, produced by Françoise Cluzeau at al. Details, availability and view instrument:
http://www.sghms.ac.uk/phs/hceu/index.htm
(121) National Guidelines Clearing House US public resource for evidence-based clinical practice guidelines:
http://www.guidelines.gov/
(122) NHS Research & Development Health Technology Assessment Programme Check publications at:
http://www.soton.ac.uk/~hta/
(123) US Health Services Technology Assessment Text Technology assessments and guidelines:
http://text.nlm.nih.gov/
(124) US National Institute for Health Consensus Statements
http://odp.od.nih.gov/consensus

Health economics

(125) Centre for Health Economics, University of York
http://www.york.ac.uk/inst/che/welcome.htm
(126) Health Economics Research Group, Brunel University Full-text Reports, links:
http://httpl.brunel.ac.uk:8080/depts/herg/
(127) Health Economics Research Centre, University of Oxford Links to health economics resources worldwide:
http://www.ihs.ox.ac.uk/herc/
(128) Health Economics Research Unit (HERU), Dept of Community Medicine, University of Aberdeen Economic appraisal methods, links to health economics research group sites:
http://www.abdn.ac.uk/public health/heru/index.html
(129) International Health Economics Association (iHEA) Excellent gateway site:
http://www.healtheconomics.org/

Health outcomes

(130) Nuffield Institute for Health, University of Leeds
  http://www.leeds.ac.uk/nuffield/home.html
  Access to several databases covering a wide range of material, including 'grey' literature:
  UK Clearing House on Health Outcomes: Databases:
    Outcomes Literature Database
    Outcomes Activities Database
    Outcomes Database of Structured Abstracts
  see also: European Clearing Houses on Health Outcomes and European Clearing House
  on Health System Reforms.

EBM Web sites

(131) Centre for Evidence-Based Child Health, Institute of Child Health
  http://www.ich.bpmf.ac.uk/ebm/ebm.htm
(132) Centre for Evidence-Based Dentistry, Institute of Health Sciences, Oxford Great links
  for dentistry and oral health:
  http://www.ihs.ox.ac.uk/cebd/index.htm
(133) Centre for Evidence-Based Medicine, Oxford University Links, news, conferences,
  learning materials, journal contents, critical appraisal software, collection of critically
  appraised topics (CATS) and more:
  http://cebm.jr2.ox.ac.uk
(134) Centre for Evidence-Based Mental Health, Institute of Health Science, Oxford
  Toolkit, links, RCPsych. Clinical guidelines, full-text articles from secondary journal
  Evidence-Based Mental Health (54); see also (107).
  http://www.psychiatry.ox.ac.uk/cebmh
(135) Centre for Evidence-Based Nursing, based at University of York Projects,
  publications, links:
  http://www.york.ac.uk/depts/hstd/centres/evidence/ev-intro.htm
(136) Evidence Based Medicine University of Hertfordshire, Learning Resource Centre:
  EBM bibliography, resources, links:
  http://www.herts.ac.uk/lrc/subjects/health/ebm.htm

Electronic journals

See also Electronic Publications on (84); use search engines to find Web sites of journal
  publishers (e.g. Health Service Journal: *http://www.hsj.macmillan.com/*). Priory Lodge Education
  produce several on-line, peer-reviewed journals, e.g. (56) above, with free registration:
  http://www.priory.com/

(137) Directory of Biomedical Journals on the Web Directory of 2800 journals on the Web,
  produced by Masaaki Tonosaki of Nippon Medical School Central Library; available via
  OMNI:
  http://omni.ac.uk/mirror/tonoej12.pdf and
  http://libserve.nms.ac.jp/ovidweb/tonoej12.pdf
(138) BioMedNet The Internet Community for Biological and Medical Researchers. Free
  registration for full-text library of 200 journals, databases (including free Medline),
  bookshop, daily research news, magazine, document delivery service, database of Internet
  Resources, shopping mall, search engine, jobs:
  http://BioMedNet.com

Databases

See Gateway sites above, also entries 94, 100, 106, 109 and 135 and entries for specific
  Databases.

(139) Dr Felix's Free Medline Page Summary chart with links to free Medline sites, bulletin board for messages and information on Internet health-care databases, news, comments, search hints:
http://www.docnet.org.uk/drfelix
(140) PubMed & Grateful Med Medline and other major databases from US National Library of Medicine:
http://www.ncbi.nlm.nih.gov/Pubmed/
(141) List of free Medline sites, some reviewed
http://omni.ac.uk/general-info/internet medicine.html
(142) Evaluation of current Web Medlines
http://omni.ac.uk/agec/iolim97/
(143) Doctors Desk Trial version of subscription search facility for clinicians:
http://www.drsdesk.sghms.ac.uk

Database and resource providers

This is the briefest selection (not endorsement) of commercial providers who offer various combinations of on-line, CD-ROM or Web access to databases and other electronic resources:

(144) Knight-Ridder Information, London DIALOG and DataStar databases on-line:
http://www.krinfo.com
(145) Ovid Technologies CD-ROM and on-line databases:
http://www.ovid.com
(146) SilverPlatter Information Ltd CD-ROM and ERL networkable databases:
http://silverplatter.com
(147) microinfo ltd Distributors of wide range of mainly CD-ROM resources:
http://www.microinfo.co.uk/

4

Introduction to critical appraisal

Martin Dawes

The aim of critical appraisal is to identify the quality of an article. There are three key issues to think about when appraising any paper:

- Are the results of the study valid?
- What are the results?
- Are the results relevant?

It can be hard to get any research published. Before the paper gets sent to a journal it will often have gone through eight or nine drafts with each author changing the contents and the appearance. The paper then arrives at the journal and is sent for a brief scrutiny. This will decide whether it then enters the process of peer review. If it passes this first scrutiny, it will be sent to several people who work in the same field for their opinion. This opinion is usually classified into several areas such as originality, statistical quality and methodological quality. The journal then decides whether to accept the paper. The reviewers will certainly have made some comments and the journal will ask the authors to rewrite the paper incorporating those comments. These may range from very minor changes to major analysis and rewrites. Finally the paper is accepted and is published.

Given this process why do we need appraisal? Surely this rigorous approach would ensure that all research published is of good quality. To begin with, there may be journals that are less rigorous in their approach to peer review. This is not the case for the majority of journals and certainly not the most prestigious journals. So why not accept research published in a major journal? The chief reason is that the reviewers may not check the methodology in a systematic way. Unlike the system described in the next few chapters, there is no standard reviewer's checklist to ensure simple research processes have been performed adequately, though individual journals may circulate their own guidance.

Is all published research flawed? The answer is categorically no. The process of designing a study and ensuring that it will answer the posed question is very time consuming and costly. Funding bodies will scrutinise research protocols before money is awarded just as rigorously as journals assess articles relating to it. However, not all research is externally funded and so may not go through this process.

In one's enthusiasm to develop an idea or share a discovery, certain factors affecting the research can be overlooked. Finally hindsight is a wonderful tool. We should not forget that the researchers are working without the benefit of this!

So how do you start? First, it may be easier to try to do it with someone else. Second, it is very hard to appraise a paper if you have not read it. That may sound obvious. When we run workshops we ask people to read a paper before the session. Very few of the tutors let alone the students have managed to find time to do this. So for any session appraising a paper always allow 10 or 15 minutes at the beginning for reading the paper. Third, start with easy questions. For example, have the authors answered the question the research was designed to study? A simple question, but often you see studies that outline a finding that was discovered by accident during the process of data collection. Fourth, do not stop appraising once you find flaws in the work. There may still be useful information in the study.

Fifth, review your appraisal. You will be amazed how easy it is to 'rubbish' a paper. You are using hindsight and tools/checklists that may have been designed after the research was published. The art of appraisal is to assess not whether the paper is 'rubbish', but whether there is so much potential bias that the results are no longer valid. That is a slightly odd sentence but does contain the essence of appraisal. Certainly when you start appraising there are many difficulties. Being unfamiliar with research papers is the first.

This all sounds like it will take far too long and be far too difficult. To start with, it will feel uncomfortable. If you think about everyday life, you are judging the information you receive all the time for its completeness and trustworthiness, in newspaper articles, for example, or information received from people you meet. Undertaking a critical appraisal is really just using your everyday skills, and applying them in a more structured and systematic way. After you have read the following chapters and you have increased your understanding, you will feel more confident and be able to start developing your skills. Once you read one or two articles a week your confidence (and speed) will pick up. Not only that, but your knowledge and practice may even change as well!

5

Randomised controlled trials

Martin Dawes

One of the best sources of information that I consult regularly is the British National Formulary (BNF). It contains most of the drugs that I use in everyday practice and I can find my way around it very easily. I use it several times each day to check dosages, side effects, drug interactions and also to review prescribing guidelines for various chronic conditions such as epilepsy. Its advantages are that the layout for each drug is similar, the book comes with a certain authority, and most UK health professionals use it. In comparison, the identification of information from a research article is much harder. The layout is frequently different depending on the journal you are reading. You are often relying on the editorial board of the journal as well as the people who reviewed the article to have ensured the quality of the article. There may be confusing statistics that make interpretation of the data seem difficult. These problems seem to be very daunting when you are trying to identify information that may affect the care of a patient.

One problem is the time it may take to read through and identify all the major features of an article. The aim of the next section is to speed up the process whilst ensuring quality. If you can assess the quality of a paper very quickly, then you can decide whether or not to continue the process of appraisal.

CONTENTS OF ARTICLES ON THERAPY

Treatment articles do not always use a consistent format when describing their results. It has taken many years for articles in scientific journals to reach a reasonably similar format of presentation. An article usually contains the following sections: abstract, introduction, methods, results, discussion and references. Even so the layout of the articles differs from journal to journal. So what information can you gather from the abstract? After all, this is the part of the article you are most likely to read (usually going directly to the last line in the conclusions section!).

A general practitioner (GP) is questioning the use of antibiotics in children with ear infections (otitis media). He designs his question and, after searching, finds this article: Burke P, Bain J, Robinson D, Dunleavey J 1991 Acute red ear in children: controlled trial of non-antibiotic treatment in general practice. British Medical Journal 303:558–562.

Objective. To examine the efficacy and safety of conservative management of mild otitis media ('the acute red ear') in children.

Here the authors clearly define that they are looking at safety as well as effectiveness of treatment. This is particularly important when comparing experimental treatment with placebo.

Design. Double blind placebo controlled trial.

Not only were the patients blind to (did not know) the treatment but the doctors were also unaware if their patient was taking experimental or placebo drugs.

Setting. 17 group general practices (48 general practitioners) in Southampton, Bristol and Portsmouth.

This describes where the study took place. It helps us decide whether the study is relevant to our practice, which may be in a different setting (see Ch. 16).

Patients. 232 children aged 3 to 10 years with acute earache and at least one abnormal eardrum (114 allocated to receive antibiotic, 118 placebo).

From Chapter 2 we know we should have a three-part question comprising (1) the patient, (2) the intervention and (3) the outcome. We can see here whether the patients in this study match those of the GP's hypothetical question.

Interventions. Amoxycillin 125 mg three times a day for 7 days or matching placebo; in addition to 100 ml paracetamol 120 mg/5 ml.

Is the intervention a practical choice for you and does it sound sensible for the patients involved?

Main outcome measures. Diary records of pain and crying, use of analgesic, eardrum signs, failure of treatment, tympanometry at 1 and 3 months, recurrence rate, and ear, nose, and throat referral rate over 1 year.

You may be concerned about the validity of diary records on pain and crying, but tympanometry probably is reliable. Are these the outcome measures that you would regard as important and relevant to your question?

Results. Treatment failure was eight times more likely in the placebo than the antibiotic group (14.4% vs 1.7%, odds ratio 8.21, 95% confidence interval 1.94 to 34.7). Children in the placebo group showed a significantly higher incidence of fever on the day after entry (20% vs 8%, p less than 0.05), mean analgesic consumption (0.36 ml/h vs 0.21 ml/h, difference 0.14, 95% confidence interval 0.07 to 0.23; $p = 0.0022$), mean duration of crying (1.44 days vs 0.50 days, 0.94; 0.50 to 1.38; p less than 0.001), and mean absence from school (1.96 days vs 0.52 days, 1.45; 0.46 to 2.42; $p = 0.0132$). Differences in recorded pain were not significant. The prevalence of middle ear effusion at 1 or 3 months, as defined by tympanometry, was not significantly different, nor was there any difference in recurrence rate or in ear, nose, and throat referral rate in the follow-up year. No characteristics could be identified which predicted an adverse outcome.

This is the stage at which many of us get confused. The first line usually contains the meat of the paper. Here the author states clearly that treatment failure was eight times more likely in the placebo than the antibiotic group. The rest of the results describes other end points of the study. If the GP's question was about the effectiveness of antibiotics in reducing crying here is the answer. However, other end points such as tympanometry at 1 month showed no difference.

Conclusions. Use of antibiotic improves short-term outcome substantially and therefore continues to be an appropriate management policy.

Finally, the authors write a conclusion that describes their opinion of the results.

Having read this synopsis, would the GP now use this treatment in his patients to reduce the duration of crying? What questions form in the GP's mind while reading the article? There is a lot of information carried in the abstract but not enough to completely check the validity of the article.

One aspect of this study was the duration of the symptoms before treatment and the authors state that the difference in duration of symptoms to entering the study was not significant. The GP may want to check this by going to the methods section:

Boys were slightly more common in the antibiotic group (59/114, 52%) than in the placebo group (50/118, 42%), but the groups did not differ in terms of age, geographical location, social class, season of entry, recorded history of otitis media, and history of ear, nose, and throat referral or ear surgery. Four children receiving antibiotic and eight placebo had had an adenoidectomy. Mean duration of pain before entry to the trial was 35.8 hours in the antibiotic group and 30.1 hours in the placebo group (difference not significant). The two groups had similar physical signs at entry, except that 19 children had one or more bulging eardrums in the antibiotic group compared with eight in the placebo group.

This shows that the duration was different but that this difference was not statistically different. The methods section should describe how the research was designed to enable the answer to be provided. This section will often be very informative to the appraiser in understanding or detecting the validity of that research.

The results section should describe clearly the demographic features of the patients in terms of age, sex and other relevant characteristics. It should then outline the specific characteristics of the problem that the research addresses, for instance the severity of the disability in whatever measure has been used. Finally, it should present in tabular form the main results of the intervention. Included in this table should be not only evidence of clinical effectiveness, but also statistical significance. This latter should enable you as a reader to determine whether this finding may have happened by chance and whether the same finding is likely to occur if the research was performed again in other populations.

So where does this leave the GP? Does he believe the results? Is the research of sufficiently good quality for him to believe? It may be helpful at this stage to introduce a list of useful questions to ask of any therapeutic article (Box 5.1). These questions are derived from several sources including what are known as the JAMA guidelines (Guyatt et al 1993).

The advantage of the BNF is that we are familiar with the layout and can quickly find the relevant information. Only by practising appraisal skills can we gain that familiarity with research papers. Chapter 3 on Finding the Evidence dealt with the types of papers that would be likely to contain information relevant to therapy. These are the questions that are important when considering a paper on therapy.

Box 5.1 Guidelines for appraising a therapeutic article

1 Did the authors answer the question?
2 Were groups of patients randomised?
3 Are the comparison groups similar?
4 Were patients blinded?
5 Was it placebo controlled?
6 Was evaluation of effect blinded?
7 Was the length of study appropriate?
8 What was the follow-up rate?
9 Are there clear measures of outcome?

   • Was it an 'intention-to-treat' trial? (See Ch. 14)
   • Is the context of the study similar to your own? (See Ch. 16)
   • Did the treatment work? (See Ch. 14)

---

1. DID THE AUTHORS ANSWER THE QUESTION?

Each article written has an introduction in which the authors put forward the context of the problem and justify their research by demonstrating the lack of evidence within the literature. At the end of this section you will often find described the exact question that the research has been designed to answer. Sometimes authors put this into the abstract while others leave it to the discussion. Finally, some authors leave you guessing as to what the original question might have been.

2. WERE THE GROUPS RANDOMISED?

The major reason for randomisation is to prevent bias. The largest potential cause of bias in research about effectiveness of an intervention is if the patients allocated to the treatment group are different from those allocated to the control group in a way that might influence outcome. To reduce this bias as much as possible, the decision as to which treatment a patient receives should be determined by random allocation. Why is this important? Consider a practitioner allocating hypertensive patients to experimental or placebo treatment. The practitioner has the patients' best outcome in mind. When patients with very high ranges of blood pressure come in he may be wary of using placebo and so allocate patients to experimental treatment, in patients with borderline hypertension, vice versa, preferring to use the placebo. If you were determining how effective the drug was in bringing people below a certain threshold, the effect of this bias would be as follows. The drug might seem not to work as well as placebo in returning patients' blood pressure below a certain threshold because more borderline patients received placebos. It is the borderline group in which you are more likely to see treatment successes, simply because it is easier to bring them below the threshold.

Alternative methods of allocation are to use the day of the week, birth date or patient identification number. These non-random methods may result in biased results. The day of the week that patients can attend the doctor varies with work and home circumstances. Thus, selecting alternate days may introduce a bias. Some diseases are related to season of birth, and high registration numbers are likely to be given to people who have recently moved into the area.

True random allocation can result in some differences occurring between the two groups through chance. This can lead to difficulty when analysing the results if, for instance, there was an important difference in severity of disease between the two groups. This can be addressed at the early stages of a study by using 'stratified randomisation'. The researcher identifies the most important factors relevant to that research question and stratifies by these factors. An example of this is an Australian hypertension study looking at the impact of the therapy on total cardiovascular events (Wing et al 1997). This study stratifies patients by age and general practice to ensure that patients in the intervention and the control groups are similar with regard to these factors

3. ARE THE COMPARISON GROUPS SIMILAR?

To determine whether bias has occurred in the selection procedure certain potentially relevant characteristics of the two populations should be displayed in tabular form. Usually these include age, sex, duration of illness and other demographic and functional characteristics. If the treatment is studying the effect of a drug on mortality, for example, then the age of the subjects in either arm of the study will have an effect on the overall rate of mortality. A paper describing two options of therapy will usually have a table describing the characteristics of each group and may evaluate whether any differences between the groups are statistically significant. For example, a study investigating the use of a cardiovascular drug might describe the characteristics as shown in Table 5.1. A brief view of this table will then enable you to ensure that the groups are similar.

Table 5.1 Characteristics of patients (n = 4230) randomised to experimental or placebo treatment

	Experimental	Placebo
Age	52.5 (52.0–53.0)	55.4 (55.1–55.8)
Male sex	51.8%	45.5%
Blue eyes	43%	65%
Mean clinic systolic BP (mmHg)	159.1(158.2–159.9)	164.1 (163.6–164.7)
Mean clinic diastolic BP (mmHg)	94.2 (93.7–94.7)	96.1 (95.9–96.3)
Cardiovascular deaths	38	33
Follow-up (months)	23.2 (22.4–24.0)	28.0 (27.6–28.5)

BP, blood pressure.

The means of these characteristics are accompanied by confidence intervals (See Ch. 14). These allow you to determine whether the two populations are truly similar. Some of these features may not be important such as the colour of the eyes in determining mortality. In that case it probably is not clinically significant. The age or the gender may be very relevant if mortality is the outcome being studied.

4. & 5. PATIENTS BLINDED AND PLACEBO-CONTROLLED

Placebos are inactive versions of the treatment. Even though they are pharmacologically inert they still have an effect on the disease (See Ch. 14, p161). Studies investigating a therapy should be designed so that the patients are unaware (single blind) of whether their treatment is experimental or placebo. If the trial is of a medication that can be given in tablet form, the pharmaceutical company involved will usually provide both placebo and experimental treatments to the researcher already packaged and sealed so that the researcher cannot know which they are giving. If there is a trial of medication that may have large cost implications, companies do not analyse the data themselves but give the analysis over to a third party such as a university department of statistics. In this way bias is excluded all the way from the clinician down to the presentation of the results.

6. BLIND ASSESSMENT

If the outcome relies on the judgement of the clinician and that clinician knows that the patient has had the experimental treatment, the clinician's interpretation of clinical findings may be exposed to bias. As researchers we put forward a hypothesis and aim to prove or disprove that hypothesis using research. Inevitably we have staked some intellectual investment in the outcome of the study and wish for a positive result. It is therefore extremely hard to be totally unbiased in the clinical evaluation of the outcome, when aware of the intervention that the patient has undergone.

This also extends to the evaluation of clinical findings recorded by others in the notes. Researchers identifying positive outcomes may search harder through the notes for an indication of that outcome if they are aware of the treatment. As a result it is preferable for clinicians to be blind in addition to the patients (double blind).

7. LENGTH OF STUDY

The length of the study is critical in determining the clinical significance of the results. For a disease of short duration, for example an acute infectious disease, the period of the study need only be long enough to cover the course of that infection. Where the disease is more progressive and lengthy, the duration of the study needs to reflect that. The question that the research is trying to answer will also be helpful in deciding the appropriate length of the study. In the example of a patient with acute painful arthritis the question might be about pain relief from that acute attack in which case the research need only be quite short. Another question might be the impact that a drug might have on the mobility of the patient following a prolonged period of treatment. This study would need to be of sufficient length to address that aspect.

A study is set up to look at the effect of antibiotics on children with ear infections. The study aims to determine whether the use of antibiotics shortens the duration of symptoms including pain and fever. The study is performed and clearly demonstrates that at 3 days antibiotics have reduced both of these characteristics. From this evidence it is clear that antibiotics have a role in the treatment of ear infections in children. However, what has not been demonstrated is that at 7 days there is no difference between the two groups in pain or fever. This further information may affect your protocol for treatment of this condition.

In order to determine the appropriate length for a study you should first have an idea of the natural progress of the disease itself.

8. FOLLOW-UP

The undertaking of a clinical trial is usually time consuming and difficult to complete properly. A good clinical trial requires the complete follow-up of patients in both the placebo and experimental treatment groups. If less than 80% of patients are adequately followed up, then the results may be invalid. To assess the thoroughness of the article check that follow-up was discussed. The American College of Physicians has decided to use 80% as its threshold for inclusion of papers into the ACP Journal and Evidence Based Medicine (ACP Journal Club 1994). If the 20% not followed up had the opposite outcome, then the overall results would be unlikely to vary substantially.

During any study it is extremely difficult to follow up all the individuals in the study. In the UK the turnover of the patient list of an average family practitioner is 7% per year; that is 7% of all registered patients each year will have moved out of the area, transferred to another practitioner or died. This indicates the difficulty in tracing patients entered into a study that lasts for anything longer than a few weeks.

The other major feature affecting the follow-up is patient compliance. A large proportion of patients may never complete the treatment. I am sure that very few of you have completed even a 5-day course of an antibiotic. Not because you suffered side effects or the treatment did not work but just because life is too hectic. It is often not convenient to attend the clinic or the hospital to have a repeat assessment of the illness and further investigations, particularly if you are feeling better.

The compliance with the quite rigorous follow-up requirements of drug trials is a major problem. Patients are not paid to be included in a study and therefore have to have some other incentive for attending. Frequently this may be a difficult illness that has not responded to current therapy. This means that those not attending may not have responded to the treatment as well as those who have responded, or vice versa.

This is the reason that researchers strive to get the maximum response rate in order to avoid bias. In calculating the results of their study researchers often will include non-attendees in the analysis by giving them the worst possible outcome studied (Schulz et al 1996). This reflects more accurately what will happen in the real world when you give a treatment rather than in some super compliant population. For a study into the role of a treatment to reduce pain from arthritis the researchers would include in the analysis the patients who had not come back for their evaluation as having the maximum pain after treatment.

9. OUTCOME MEASURES

To determine the impact of an intervention on patient health you need to define clearly the outcome that needs to be measured. This sounds straightforward enough but can take up a larger amount of the preparation time of the research. What is meant by outcome measure?

An outcome measure is any feature that is recorded to determine the progression of the disease or problem being studied. A large number of studies are undertaken to evaluate the impact of therapies on arthritis. The outcome measure that is presented in the paper may not be the most relevant to the patients. Restriction in mobility may be of more importance than the presence or severity of pain although both are clearly related. Thus, a paper only describing pain relief may not necessarily have answered the question about mobility. As researchers we often assume the most important clinical features of a disease which may not be the same as those most relevant to the day-to-day lives of our patients. It is one of the reasons that qualitative research is so important in determining what is relevant to the patient.

When the outcome measure being used in the research appears appropriate, examine the thresholds of that measure used to determine severity. In terms of ability to walk we may ask patients how far they can walk or we may give them options such as 50 yards, 100 yards or 150 yards. The researcher may then make an arbitrary decision that the ability to walk 1 mile is the aim of the therapy. The researcher will then present results in terms of how many patients reached that threshold. Another question might be about the assessment of the distance walked. Was it the patient or clinician judging it, or was there an objective measurement? What is not so desirable is the researcher who finds that the therapy is effective in enabling patients to walk $\frac{1}{2}$ a mile, but not 1 mile and so uses $\frac{1}{2}$ mile retrospectively as the threshold for improvement. It is difficult, if not impossible, to detect whether this has taken place. Critical appraisers will determine what threshold they would have used for walking distance and see whether the one used in the paper approximates to their own choice.

Other authors will describe the mean walking distance before and after treatment. They can then describe statistical significant improvements in walking distance. What this description does not tell you is the number of patients who have improved. The use of means or averages hides important information about the characteristics of patients who have improved and perhaps more importantly, those who have got worse. The presentation of data is therefore critical to the use of a paper. When examining a paper in detail, check back to the introduction and title to determine whether the author really has addressed the problem properly in the results.

SUMMARY

Although this may seem very complicated, it can be broken down into manageable chunks. To start appraising for the first time, try working with two or three other people. Look at each of the questions described above relating to a paper you have chosen and write down your comments, for example

1. Follow-up was 78%. Is this high enough?

Complete all the questions. At the beginning of appraisal many people new to it are surprised at the number of flaws in papers even from established journals. It is therefore quite easy to 'rubbish' a paper. This will give you confidence to begin with. The skill of appraisal is not only to answer these quality questions, but then to go on to evaluate how these flaws might influence the results. Would 78% follow-up significantly alter the results in this paper? By examining critically you seek to assess the inference of bias produced during the research, on the eventual results. It is quite possible to value and use results from research that does contain bias. That is the real skill of appraisal.

REFERENCES

ACP Journal Club 1994 120(3): A9–10

Burke P, Bain J, Robinson D, Dunleavey J 1991 Acute red ear in children: controlled trial of non-antibiotic treatment in general practice. British Medical Journal, 303:558–562

Guyatt G, Sackett D, Cook D 1993 Users' guides to the medical literature. II. How to use an article about therapy or prevention. A. Are the results of the study valid? Evidence-Based Medicine Working Group. Journal of the American Medical Association 270:2598–2601

Schulz K, Grimes D, Altman D, Hayes R 1996 Blinding and exclusions after allocation in randomised controlled trials: survey of published parallel group trials in obstetrics and gynaecology. British Medical Journal 312:742–744

Wing L, Reid C, Ryan P et al 1997 Second Australian National Blood Pressure study (ANBP2). Australian comparative outcome trial of ACE inhibitor- and diuretic-based treatment of hypertension in the elderly. Management Committee on behalf of the High Blood Pressure Research Council of Australia. Clinical Experimental Hypertension 19:779–791

6

Studies assessing diagnostic tests

Jonathan Mant

Diagnoses are usually made through interpreting and combining information from a combination of the clinical history, examination findings and the results of investigations such as blood tests and X-rays. An important component of evidence-based health care is working out how useful these different pieces of information are in making a diagnosis. For example, if you test a patient's urine and find protein in it, how likely is it that this represents kidney disease? Or if you find sugar in it, how likely is it that the patient has diabetes? A test result needs to be interpreted in the light of how accurate you think the test is, and what you already know about the patient. We will look at how to combine your knowledge about the test and the patient in Chapter 13. In this chapter, we consider the types of studies that are carried out to assess how good a test is, and how to critically appraise them.

What is meant by test accuracy? Usually, this is expressed in terms of the sensitivity and specificity of the test. Sensitivity reflects the ability of a test to identify people who have disease and specificity reflects the ability of the test to identify 'normality', or people who do not have disease. These terms are discussed in greater detail in Chapter 13, together with other terms that are also used to summarise test accuracy such as predictive value and likelihood ratio. Here, we are concerned with how a study might be done to assess the accuracy of a test. To illustrate the principles, we will use a specific example, namely a study performed to assess how good is clinical assessment at making a diagnosis of deep vein thrombosis (DVT) (Wells et al 1995).

EXAMPLE: STUDY TO ASSESS ACCURACY OF CLINICAL ASSESSMENT OF DEEP VEIN THROMBOSIS

In this study, Wells et al wanted to find out how useful clinical history and examination are in making the diagnosis of DVT. The patients in the study were those who had been referred to out-patient clinics in three hospitals (two in Canada and one in Italy) for the evaluation of suspected DVT. Out of 887 consecutive patients who were referred for this reason to these hospitals, 529 were included in the study. In the out-patient clinics, patients were seen by physicians who regularly assess people for this problem. The clinicians summarised their clinical assessment by categorising the patients into three groups: high, moderate and low probability of DVT. This was done by looking for explicit features in the history and examination (Table 6.1), and considering whether or not there was an alternative diagnosis. Patients were assessed as having a high probability of DVT if they had no alternative diagnosis and either at least three major points or two major and two minor points suggestive of DVT (Table 6.1). Other possible combinations of major and minor points and presence or absence of alternative diagnoses were assessed as being of moderate or low probability of DVT according to an explicit scoring system (Wells et al 1995). Venograms were then performed on all the patients. Venography is generally recognised to be the most accurate way to make the diagnosis. The results were interpreted by a panel of at least three observers who were unaware of the patient's clinical history and of the results of any other diagnostic test (in this study, most of the patients also had ultrasound).

The results are analysed by comparing those obtained by the diagnostic test(s) being evaluated (in this case, clinical assessment) with a 'reference standard' test (in this case, venography). An ideal reference standard test (see below) is one which always gives the correct answer. In other words, it always tells the truth. The result of the comparison of clinical assessment with venography is shown in Table 6.2. This shows, if we accept that the venogram is always right, that 26% of the patients referred with suspected DVT actually turned out to have one. It also shows that clinical assessment was by no means perfect. Some patients (n = 16) who were thought to have a low probability of DVT turned out to have DVT, and some patients who were thought to have a high probability of DVT (n = 13) did not have one. Nevertheless, the clinical assessment did reasonably well, in that someone assessed as having a high probability of DVT actually turned out to have an 85% chance of having DVT. Likewise, someone assessed as having a low probability of DVT did indeed have a low probability of having a positive

Table 6.1 Features of history and examination used in clinical assessment of DVT

	History	Examination
Major points	Active cancer Paresis or immobilisation of legs Recently bedridden (>3 days) or major surgery within 4 weeks Strong family history of DVT	Local tenderness along deep venous system distribution Swelling of thigh and calf
Minor points	Recent injury of symptomatic leg Hospitalisation within 6 months	Pitting oedema only on symptomatic leg Dilated superficial veins only on symptomatic leg Erythema

Adapted from Wells et al (1995).

Table 6.2 Comparison of clinical assessment of DVT with venography in 529 patients with suspected DVT

| | Venography result | | |
	Positive (%)	Negative	Totals
Clinical assessment			
High probability of DVT	72 (85)	13	85
Moderate probability of DVT	47 (33)	96	143
Low probability of DVT	16 (5)	285	301
Totals	135 (26)	394	529

Adapted from Wells et al (1995).

venogram (5%). Formally, the accuracy of clinical assessment of DVT can be summarised using a number of different terms, as shown in Table 6.3. The significance and meaning of these terms is described in Chapter 13.

However, it is important not to just take the results of a study at face value, but to decide for yourself whether or not you think the study was sufficiently well performed that you can trust its results. There are specific criteria which can be used against which the validity of a study assessing the value of a diagnostic test can be measured (Jaeschke et al 1994). We will now consider what these criteria mean, and consider them in terms of the DVT study.

1. WAS THE REFERENCE STANDARD APPROPRIATE?

To start with, we need to find out how the study found out what the 'truth' really was about patients. That is to say, how did the investigators know whether or not someone really had a disease? To do this, they will have needed some reference standard test (or series of tests) which they know 'always' tells the truth.

Examples of reference standards that have been used to assess some diagnostic tests are shown in Table 6.4. Sometimes, there may not be a single test that is suitable as a reference standard. In such situations, a battery of tests may need to be performed, and an 'expert' panel may need to decide whether disease is present or absent. For example, in the study by

Table 6.3 Summary measures of accuracy of clinical assessment of DVT as compared to venography

Sensitivity	72/135	53%
Specificity	381/394	97%
Positive predictive value	72/85	85%
Negative predictive value	381/444	86%
Likelihood ratio (+ve)	0.533/(1 − 0.967)	16.1
Likelihood ratio (−ve)	(1 − 0.53)/0.97	0.5

Calculations are done for clinical assessment of 'high probability' of DVT.
Calculated from data provided by Wells et al (1995).
See example at end of Chapter 13 for further details of calculation.

Table 6.4   Examples of diagnostic tests and possible reference standards

Diagnostic test	Reference standard	Reference
Mammography for breast cancer	Biopsy for test positives; clinical follow-up for test negatives	UK Trial of Early Detection of Breast Cancer Group (1992)
Doppler ultrasonography for carotid artery stenosis	Carotid arteriogram	Carpenter et al (1995)
Urinalysis using test strip for urinary tract infections	Culture of urine in the laboratory	Winkens et al (1995)
Electrocardiograph for diagnosing heart failure	Echocardiography	Davie et al (1996)
Magnetic resonance imaging for multiple sclerosis (MS)	Review by panel of two neurologists specialising in MS and a neuroradiologist of: —clinical history, examination findings, and follow-up —all laboratory and neurophysiological tests	Mushlin et al (1993)
Ventilation/perfusion (V/Q) scan for pulmonary embolus	Pulmonary angiogram or clinical follow-up for 1 year	PIOPED Investigators (1990)

Mushlin et al (1993) of the accuracy of magnetic resonance imaging (MRI) for the diagnosis of multiple sclerosis, a single reference standard could not be used since there is no perfect test for multiple sclerosis. Instead, Mushlin et al asked a panel of experts to review all the clinical data about the patients, with the exception, of course, of the MRI result! Included in this data was follow-up information concerning any clinical developments after the patients had their MRI scan.

Sometimes, it is not possible to carry out the same reference standard test for all the patients in the study. For example, the PIOPED investigators (1990) used two reference standards in their assessment of ventilation/perfusion (V/Q) scanning as a test for pulmonary embolus. They used pulmonary angiography or they used clinical follow-up for 12 months. Pulmonary angiography is highly accurate and is the recognised reference standard for this diagnosis. However, it is an invasive investigation with a risk of complications. It is difficult to justify on ethical grounds carrying out this investigation on people who you do not think have had a pulmonary embolus, such as those in the study with a normal V/Q scan. Therefore, the PIOPED investigators used a different reference standard for those patients in whom pulmonary angiography could not be performed. They followed them up for 12 months without treatment for pulmonary embolus, and observed whether any of them developed any clinical evidence of pulmonary embolus. Similarly, it would have been neither ethical nor practical for the UK Breast Cancer Group (1992) in their assessment of the accuracy of mammography as a screening test for breast cancer to carry out their reference standard investigation (breast biopsy) on women who had a normal mammogram. Instead, they classified 'interval cancers' – i.e. cancers occurring within 12 months after the screening – in patients who had a normal mammogram as evidence of a false negative result.

When considering the validity of a study looking at a diagnostic test, you need to consider whether the reference standard used is sufficiently accurate, i.e. that it gives a good approximation to the truth. If it does not reflect the truth, then the results of the study will be difficult to interpret. In the DVT study, the reference standard was venography. This is the generally accepted reference standard. It is accurate, but has problems of expense, invasiveness and risk of complications, and it is not technically possible to carry out on every patient (Anand et al 1998). Nevertheless, in this context, 'appropriateness' is essentially about accuracy, so the venogram can be taken to be an appropriate reference standard.

2. WERE THE REFERENCE STANDARD AND THE DIAGNOSTIC TEST INTERPRETED INDEPENDENTLY OF EACH OTHER?

If the study investigators know what the result of the reference standard is, this might influence their interpretation of the diagnostic test and vice versa. Suppose we wanted to evaluate how good auscultation (listening with a stethoscope) of the chest is to diagnose pneumonia. A simple reference standard we could use might be a chest X-ray. It is much easier to hear crackles in the chest if we have seen changes on the X-ray, and we might be more likely to consider a chest X-ray abnormal if we knew that there were abnormalities on auscultation. Therefore, to ensure that the results of one test are not influenced by the results of the other test, it is important that each is carried out independently of the other. The person interpreting one test should be blind to (i.e. does not know) the results of the other test.

In the study of the accuracy of clinical assessment of DVT, the clinical assessments were carried out before the venograms, and the venograms were interpreted without knowledge of the clinical assessment (Wells et al 1995). Therefore, in this example, the reference standard and the diagnostic test were indeed interpreted independently of each other.

3. WAS THE REFERENCE STANDARD APPLIED TO ALL PATIENTS?

Ideally, both the test being evaluated and the reference standard should be carried out on all patients in the study. However, this may not be possible for both practical and ethical reasons, as was discussed above. In many cases, the reference standard test may be invasive and may expose the patient to some risk and/or discomfort. While it would usually be ethical to use such a test in a patient in whom you had grounds to suspect that it might be positive, it would not be ethical if you thought that the test would be negative (i.e. if the diagnostic test being evaluated had been negative). Therefore, when reading the paper you need to find out whether the reference standard was applied to all patients, and if it was not, look at what steps the investigators took to find out what the 'truth' was in patients who did not have the reference test. Examples have been given above – pulmonary angiography as a reference standard for pulmonary embolus, and biopsy for breast cancer – where it is not possible to carry out the preferred reference standard on all patients. In each of these cases, the studies cited followed up their patients for a period of time to see if any signs of the disease developed as an alternative.

In the study by Wells et al (1995), 635 patients were in fact eligible for the study, but only 529 patients had the reference standard applied. This was either because patients did not give consent to take part in the study, or because a venogram could not be performed. Rather than use an alternative reference standard, the investigators excluded patients who did not have venograms from the study. Since their exclusion was not on the basis of the clinical assessment of probability of DVT, this is not a serious problem.

4. WAS THE TEST EVALUATED ON THE RIGHT SORT OF PATIENTS?

Another complication is that a test may perform differently depending upon the sort of patients on whom it is carried out. For example, the more severe a disease is, the easier it tends to be to detect. Thus, you might find that testing for protein in the urine might be better at detecting kidney disease when evaluated in patients who attend a renal clinic, than in those attending a general practice surgery. This is because people with kidney disease who attend a renal clinic in general will be more symptomatic and lose more protein in the urine, making it easier to detect. This problem is referred to as *spectrum bias* (see Ch. 13 for more explanation). A test is going to perform better in terms of detecting people with disease (i.e. higher sensitivity) if it is used to identify it in people in whom the disease is more severe, or advanced. Similarly, the test will produce more false positive results (i.e. have lower specificity) if it is carried out on patients with other diseases that might mimic the disease that is being tested for.

The issue to consider when appraising a paper is whether the test was evaluated on the typical sort of patients in whom the test would be carried out in real life. For example, it would not make a lot of sense to evaluate a diagnostic test on someone who you already know has the disease, since this would not be done in clinical practice – if you know they have the disease, then there is no point in carrying out further tests!

The patients in the study by Wells et al (1995) were the right sort of patients in that they did not include patients with already proven DVT, and all the patients in the study had been referred for assessment because of suspected DVT. An issue to consider here is the selection of patients for the study. Only 72% (635/887) of patients referred with suspected DVT were considered eligible for the study, and only 60% (529/887) were actually included in the study. It is important to scrutinise the reasons for their exclusion to see if they might have resulted in spectrum bias. The principal reasons for exclusion were previous history of DVT or pulmonary embolism, and clinical findings not compatible with DVT; the reasons for non-participation of eligible patients were lack of consent and inability to carry out venography. These explanations are not directly related to severity of disease or risk of false positives, so spectrum bias is unlikely to have been introduced.

5. IS IT CLEAR HOW THE TEST WAS CARRIED OUT?

To be able to apply the results of the study to your own clinical practice, you need to be confident that the test is performed in the same way in your setting as it was in the study. In the study by Wells et al (1995), 'clinical assessment' was not left as an implicit judgement, but clearly defined criteria were written down as to what constituted high, moderate and low probability of DVT. Therefore, it should be feasible to use the same clinical model in your own practice and achieve similar results.

6. IS THE TEST RESULT REPRODUCIBLE?

This is essentially asking whether you get the same result if different people carry out the test, or if the test is carried out at different times on the same person. Many studies will assess this by having different observers perform the test, and measuring the agreement between them by means of a kappa statistic. The kappa statistic takes into account the amount of agreement that you would expect by chance. For example, if two observers make a diagnosis simply by tossing a coin, you would expect them to agree for 50% of patients. A kappa score of 0 indicates no more agreement than you would expect by chance, a negative score less agreement, and a positive score, more agreement than you would expect by chance. Perfect agreement would give a score of 1. Generally, a kappa score greater than 0.60 indicates good agreement (Altman 1991).

If agreement between observers is poor, then this will undermine the utility of the test. The extent to which the test result is reproducible or not may to some extent depend upon how explicit the guidance is for how the test should be carried out (see 5. above). It may also depend upon the experience and expertise of the observer. If the test is found to have poor reproducibility, then it is likely that this will be reflected in poor test accuracy in terms of sensitivity and specificity.

Wells et al (1995) repeated the clinical assessment of 34 of their patients by a different clinician on the same day as the original assessment. They reported that the level of agreement was 'excellent' (kappa = 0.85).

CONCLUSION

When considering a study assessing a diagnostic test, it is important to decide whether or not you think the results of the study will be valid. In this chapter, we have explored a series of questions (summarised in Box 6.1) to ask of the study. The most important question is the first one: was the reference standard appropriate? If the answer to this is 'no', then the study will be very difficult to interpret. If you can answer 'yes' to all the other questions, then you can think about what the results mean, and how they might be applied to your patients (see Ch. 13). However, no study is perfect, and if the answer to one or more of the questions is 'no' (apart from the first one), this does not mean that you should automatically throw the study away. Rather, the results need to be interpreted in the light of the bias(es) that might have been introduced.

Box 6.1 Questions about the validity of studies evaluating diagnostic tests

1. Was the reference standard appropriate?
2. Were the reference standard and the diagnostic test interpreted independently of each other?
3. Was the reference standard applied to all patients?
4. Was the test evaluated on the right sort of patients?
5. Is it clear how the test was carried out?
6. Is the test result reproducible?

(Adapted from Jaeschke et al (1994).

REFERENCES

Altman D G 1991 Practical statistics for medical research. Chapman & Hall, London, p 403–409
Anand S S, Wells P S, Hunt D et al 1998 Does this patient have deep vein thrombosis? Journal of the American Medical Association 279:1094–1099
Carpenter J P, Lexa F J, Davis J T 1995 Determination of sixty percent or greater carotid artery stenosis by duplex doppler ultrasonography. Journal of Vascular Surgery 22:697–705
Davie A P, Francies C M, Love M P et al 1996 Value of the electrocardiogram in identifying heart failure due to left ventricular systolic dysfunction. British Medical Journal 312:222
Jaeschke R, Guyatt G, Sackett D L for the Evidence Based Medicine Working Group 1994 Users' guides to the medical literature III. How to use an article about a diagnostic test: A. Are the results of the study valid? Journal of the American Medical Association 271:389–391

Mushlin A I, Detsky A S, Phelps C E et al 1993 The accuracy of magnetic resonance imaging in patients with suspected multiple sclerosis. Journal of the American Medical Association 269:3146–3151

PIOPED Investigators 1990 Value of ventilation/perfusion scan in acute pulmonary embolism: results of the Prospective Investigation of Pulmonary Embolism Diagnosis (PIOPED). Journal of the American Medical Association 263:2753–2759

United Kingdom Trial of Early Detection of Breast Cancer Group 1992 Specificity of screening in United Kingdom trial of early detection of breast cancer. British Medical Journal 304:346–349

Wells P S, Hirsh J, Anderson D R et al 1995 Accuracy of clinical assessment of deep-vein thrombosis. Lancet 345:1326–1330

Winkens R A G, Leffers P, Trienekens T A M, Stobberingh E E 1995 The validity of urine examination for urinary tract infections in general practice. Family Practice 11:290–293

7

Case series and reports

Martin Dawes

Not all evidence comes from neatly packaged meta-analyses or randomised controlled trials. The initial discovery may have been one or two cases where an observant health professional started questioning. These questions may have been published as observations. These papers are 'case reports'. If several cases have been observed to show the same features, then they may be published as a case series.

How then does one assess the validity of a case or case series report? An example of a case report is shown below (Grimson T 1977 Reactions to cimetidine [letter]. Lancet: (8016): 858 © by The Lancet Ltd).

Reactions to cimetidine

Sir, I wish to report the two cases of a possible reaction to cimetidine. A 50-year-old man was admitted with acute exacerbation of pain due to reflux oesophagitis. 2 days after admission cimetidine was started at 200 mg three times daily and 400 mg at bedtime. He was discharged 9 days later and inadvertently given two bottles, one labelled cimetidine and the other labelled Tagamet (trade name of cimetidine). The instructions on each bottle were to take three tablets per day with meals and two at bedtime, so he took double doses of cimetidine for 48 hours. He felt light-headed and dizzy and noticed some pain down the right side of his neck. He started sweating profusely together with flushing and was mentally confused. The symptoms disappeared 24 hours after he reverted to a normal dose.

A 54-year-old man was admitted with an acute exacerbation of pain due to reflux oesophagitis of some 3 years duration. 2 days after admission cimetidine 200 mg was given three times per day with meals and two other tablets at bedtime. After he had been on treatment for 4 days he was told that a patient had accidentally taken double the dose resulting in symptoms, but he was not told the nature of the reaction. He was asked whether he would take a double dose to see what happened, and this he did. 24 hours later he became dizzy, drowsy, and confused with flushing and sweating. The double dose was reduced to the original dose and his symptoms gradually disappeared, and 24 hours after reduction of the dose he was normal. He had no memory for the event.

Cimetidine is said to be well tolerated, but some patients may get diarrhoea, muscular pain, rash, and dizziness. No other drugs of significance were taken by either patient. Dr Y of Company Z tells me that double doses had been taken during some clinical trials without these side effects.

This letter was written on the basis of only really one case of confusion and other symptoms arising from an excessive dose of this drug. The doctor had then confirmed the finding in a second patient and reported the finding.

What are the important features of this letter that help the reader decide whether these cases are important (see Box 7.1)?

Box 7.1   Main features of a case report

- Age
- Diagnosis
- Symptoms
- Treatment
- Dosage
- Duration
- Onset of event
- Duration of event
- Outcome of event
- Action taken during course of event
- Author origin (i.e. rival drug company!)

Not only has this doctor described all these factors but he has also gone on to repeat the increased dosage. The details he has given allow the reader to make an informed opinion of the case. There is no degree of analysis of the pharmacological cause of the mental disturbance nor any suggestion of bias. The plain facts are displayed. So how does this differ from a case series?

2 years later a case series was published in the Lancet (Schentag et al 1979). It first described 15 cases of confusion associated with cimetidine. It then described the mental state of 36 elderly ill patients on cimetidine with their levels of cimetidine in the bloodstream. The article describes 6 of the 36 patients as having severe mental reactions. It demonstrated that all 6 patients had concentrations of cimetidine that were greater then $1.25\ \mu g/ml$, whereas only 2 of the non-confused patients had levels above this threshold.

So what characteristics were important in determining the quality of this research? Some of the questions (see Box 7.2) are similar to those in appraising other sorts of trials.

In this study the authors have raised the awareness of this drug's potential for causing confusion while admitting that their patients had

---

Box 7.2   Guidelines for appraising a treatment trial

- Were all patients accounted for at the end of the study?
- Were the characteristics of the patients described fully?
- Was the treatment of all patients consistent?
- Were evaluations of symptoms or clinical findings blinded?
- Were the methods used for measurement of symptoms or clinical findings valid?
- Were the results consistent (in this case was there a dose–response, i.e. the higher the level in the bloodstream, the more likely that there was confusion)?
- Was there potential for bias (recruitment of more severely ill or confused patients)?

---

multiple health problems and were elderly. The next step was a review of the literature that took place in 1991 (Cantu & Korek 1991). The limitations of case series and case reports are many. It is very difficult to be at all certain that what you are observing is not associated with a totally different action than the one that has been suspected. Most clinicians will start to suspect abnormality when several cases occur.

In the case of AIDS this occurred after the admission of a few, young, previously fit men into hospital in California with life-threatening, immune-related disorders. These were reported in two small articles describing three cases and then another four cases in 1981. The next event was the publication of three case series together in the New England Journal of Medicine in December 1981 (Gottlieb et al 1981, Masur et al 1981, Siegal et al 1981). An epidemic was declared after 26 cases were described. This shows the rapid publication of information about potentially serious conditions. Although we may be frustrated about the time that it takes for certain information to reach the light of day, in this case at least the delay was minimal.

The data contained in case reports must always be evaluated on the basis of the scientific evidence that they are presenting. Does the observation match the data presented? The examples I have cited are well known and often used as illustrations describing the history of discovery. However, many case reports and case series have not led to eventual discoveries. Case series and case reports have to be examined very critically even when all the above criteria have been met.

REFERENCES

Cantu T, Korek J 1991 Central nervous system reactions to histamine-2 receptor blockers. Annals of Internal Medicine 114(12):1027–1034

Gottlieb M, Schroff R, Schanker H, Weisman J, Fan P, Wolf R et al 1981 *Pneumocystis carinii* pneumonia and mucosal candidiasis in previously healthy homosexual men: evidence of a new acquired cellular immunodeficiency. New England Journal of Medicine 305(24):1425–1431

Grimson T 1977 Reactions to cimetidine [letter]. Lancet i(8016):858

Masur H, Michelis M, Greene J, Onorato I, Stouwe R, Holzman R et al 1981 An outbreak of community-acquired *Pneumocystis carinii* pneumonia: initial manifestation of cellular immune dysfunction. New England Journal of Medicine 305(24):1431–1438

Schentag J, Cerra F, Calleri G, DeGlopper E, Rose J, Bernhard H 1979 Pharmacokinetic and clinical studies in patients with cimetidine-associated mental confusion. Lancet i(8109):177–181

Siegal F, Lopez C, Hammer G, Brown A, Kornfeld S, Gold J et al 1981 Severe acquired immunodeficiency in male homosexuals, manifested by chronic perianal ulcerative herpes simplex lesions. New England Journal of Medicine 305(24):1439–1444

8

Case control studies

Jonathan Mant

The two major types of observational study that are used in epidemiology are case control studies and cohort studies. In this chapter, we shall illustrate the principles of critical appraisal of an observational study by focusing on case control studies.

As discussed in Chapter 2, clinical questions can be characterised as having three or four elements: a patient, an outcome, an intervention and possibly a comparison intervention. In Chapter 3, these questions were characterised into different types, such as those concerning effectiveness, prognosis and harm. While case control and cohort studies have been used to answer questions of effectiveness, for example in the field of cancer screening (Connor et al 1991), their role in addressing questions of this type is dwarfed by the randomised controlled trial (see Ch. 5). This is because randomisation is the best technique to eliminate bias that arises from *confounding* (see below). Case control and cohort studies come into their own when the question involves harm. For example, does air pollution cause or worsen asthma in children? Does eating meat increase the risk of cancer? This is because it is usually neither feasible nor ethical to conduct a randomised controlled trial to answer this sort of question, so alternative designs must be used. Cohort studies are also of particular value in addressing questions of prognosis and natural history. For example, what is the chance that someone who is HIV positive will develop AIDS in a given period of time?

In a cohort study that is concerned with addressing questions of harm, people will be classified on the basis of their exposure to the agent under investigation and followed up over time to see if they develop the disease or diseases of interest. For example, Vessey et al (1989) were interested in looking at the health effects of oral contraception. They recruited over 17 000 women who attended Family Planning Clinics between 1968 and 1974, and followed them up for over 20 years. They classified the women in terms of the type of contraception they were using at entry to the study, and found that there was no increased mortality in users of oral contraceptives as compared to users of other forms of contraception.

In a case control study, two groups of people are identified: people who have the disease of interest ('cases'), and people who do not ('controls'). For both groups of people, exposure to the relevant risk factor (e.g. air pollution, meat consumption) is measured, and the extent to which one group is exposed is compared to the other group. For example, Feeney et al (1997) were interested in exploring whether measles vaccination in childhood might be associated with the subsequent development of inflammatory bowel disease in adulthood.

EXAMPLE: CASE CONTROL STUDY TO ASSESS WHETHER MEASLES VACCINATION IS ASSOCIATED WITH LATER DEVELOPMENT OF INFLAMMATORY BOWEL DISEASE

In this study, Feeney et al identified 164 patients from hospital records in East Dorset with a proven diagnosis of inflammatory bowel disease born in or after 1968. These patients constituted the 'cases'. They then chose two patients who did not have inflammatory bowel disease for each 'case'. These patients constituted the controls. They were selected from the same practice as each case, and were *matched* (see below) for sex and year of birth. Next, the vaccine history for both cases and controls was obtained from the general practice records, and the community health vaccination records. For the cases, if it was not possible to obtain adequate information from these sources, documentary evidence was sought from the patients themselves. For the controls, if the information was inadequate a new matched control was substituted.

The principal analysis involved the calculation of an *odds ratio*, which compares the odds that cases received measles vaccination with the odds that controls received measles vaccination. In this study, the odds ratio was 0.97, which is very near to 1. What this means is that the risk of inflammatory bowel disease was not affected by whether or not an individual had been vaccinated. If the odds ratio had been significantly greater than one, then this would have suggested that there was an association between measles vaccination and inflammatory bowel disease. If the odds ratio had been significantly less than one, this would have suggested that there was a negative association – that is, that vaccination appeared to protect against inflammatory bowel disease. The derivation of an odds ratio is shown in Box 8.1. The conclusion of the authors was that this study provided no evidence of any link between measles vaccination in early childhood and subsequent risk of inflammatory bowel disease.

In deciding how much weight to attach to this conclusion, it is important to consider how well you think the study has been performed. There are three key issues to think about when appraising any paper:

- Are the results of the study valid?
- What are the results?
- Are the results relevant?

For a case control study, these key questions can be sub-divided into eight more detailed questions, as shown in Box 8.2.

Box 8.1(a) Derivation of an odds ratio

The results of a case control study can be summarised by means of a two-by-two table:

	Cases	Controls
Exposed	a	b
Not exposed	c	d
Totals	a+c	b+d

The odds of disease (i.e. being a case) in people exposed is given by a/b.

The odds of disease in people not exposed is given by c/d.

Therefore, the odds ratio is given by a/b ÷ c/d (which is the same as ad/bc).

Using the example in the text, cases would have been patients with inflammatory bowel disease (IBD), and 'exposed' would have meant that they had received measles vaccination (MV). Thus, the results of the Feeney et al (1997) study might have looked like the following two-by-two table.

Box 8.1(b)

	IBD	Controls
Given MV	79	160
Not given MV	61	120
Totals	140	280

The odds of IBD in people given MV is 79/160, and the odds of IBD in people not given MV is 61/120. Therefore, the odds ratio is 79/160 ÷ 61/120, or (79 × 120) ÷ (61 × 160), which comes to: 0.97.

In fact, this is the same result as was given by Feeney et al, but this is a coincidence! In the published study, the data was analysed to take account of the matched design, and a crude odds ratio as was calculated above was not reported. The actual numbers of patients in each category were not given in Feeney et al, so this table is estimated from data provided in the paper.

---

1. Have potential confounding factors been identified and dealt with appropriately?

A confounding factor is something that is associated with exposure to the risk factor under study and that independently affects the risk of developing disease (Hennekens & Buring 1987). For example, in a case control study to look at whether there was an association between use of third generation oral contraceptives and risk of venous thromboembolism, potential confounders included age, smoking and use of alcohol (Spitzer et al 1996). Each of these factors is likely to be associated with both use of oral contraception and risk of venous thromboembolism (Fig. 8.1). If you do not

---

Box 8.2   Critical appraisal of a case control study

Are the results valid?
1. Have potential confounding factors been identified and dealt with appropriately?
2. Is it likely that there is bias in either the selection of the cases or in the selection of the controls?
3. Was information on exposure obtained in a way likely to be free from bias?
What are the results?
4. What is the size of the odds ratio?
5. How large are the confidence intervals around the odds ratio?
Are the results relevant?
6. Is it likely, if an association is observed, that the relationship between exposure and disease is causal?
7. How big is the risk?
8. Is exposure of patients in the study similar to the exposure of your own patients?

---

take account of these factors in some way, you cannot be sure that any association you observe between third generation oral contraceptives and venous thromboembolism is not due to the influence of the confounder, rather than an effect of oral contraception. For example, smoking is a risk factor for thromboembolism. Furthermore, it was demonstrated in the 1970s that women who take oral contraceptives are more likely to smoke than women who use other forms of contraception (Vessey et al 1976).

Therefore, an observed association between use of oral contraception and thromboembolism might be explained by smoking, since you would expect cases to be more likely than controls to be using oral contraceptives simply because they are also more likely than controls to be smokers. If this is the case, then smoking is confounding any relationship there might be between oral contraception and thromboembolism. In this example, smoking would be exaggerating any positive association that might exist between exposure and disease. However, nowadays women who take oral contraception are advised not to smoke. Therefore, it might be that, currently, users of oral contraceptives are in fact less likely to smoke than users of other forms of contraception. If this is true, then smoking would still confound any relationship between oral contraception and throm-boembolism, but the effect would be quite the opposite, in that it would disguise rather than exaggerate any association that might exist between exposure and disease.[1] In other words, confounding can work in two ways: it can cause an apparent relationship between a risk factor and a disease when there is not one, or it can conceal a real association.

Confounding can be taken into account either in the design or in the analysis of a case control study, as shown in Table 8.1. In the study by

---

[1] To distinguish between these opposite effects of confounding, sometimes the terms 'positive' and 'negative' confounding are used. Unfortunately, there is no consistency in the literature as to which is which!

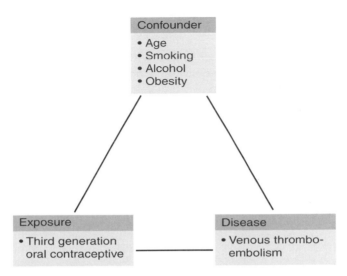

Figure 8.1   Potential confounding in a study of risk of thromboembolism in users of third generation oral contraceptives.

Feeney et al, a *matched* design was used. What this means is that for each case, the controls (two per case in this study) are specially selected to 'match' the case for the confounding factor. In this study, matching was for age, sex, and general practice. Thus, if a case was a 25-year-old man, then two controls would be selected who were also male, of the same age and from the same general practice as the case. What one needs to consider is whether it is plausible that other confounding factors might have had an effect on the result. Here, it helps if you have some knowledge about the disease being studied, and in particular, what are known risk factors. For example, the *Oxford Textbook of Medicine* lists the risk factors for Crohn's disease as time (rise in incidence since 1950), age (most common in young adults), smoking and diet (Jewell 1996). Time and age have been taken into account by the matching process, but not possible differences in smoking and diet. This does not matter unless smoking and diet are also related to whether or not measles immunisation was received, in which case they might be acting as confounders.

The other strategy for dealing with confounding in the design of a case control study is to *restrict* the cases and controls to nullify the effects of the

Table 8.1   Strategies to deal with confounding in a case control study

Design	Analysis
Restriction	Stratification
Matching	Multivariate analysis

confounder. For example, if sex was a confounder, one could remove the effect of sex if all the cases and controls were of the same gender. Feeney et al partially adopted this strategy to deal with time as a confounder in that only cases and controls born on or after 1968 were included in the study.

Alternatively, one can deal with confounding in the analysis of the case control study, either by *stratification* or *multivariate analysis*. It is beyond the scope of this book to give details of these techniques. In essence, their purpose is to derive an odds ratio that has been adjusted to take account of confounding factors. Thus, in a case control study looking at risk factors for cot death, the crude (i.e unadjusted) odds ratio for cot death where the baby slept under a duvet was 2.8. However, if the results were adjusted for confounding factors such as maternal age and birthweight, the odds ratio fell to 1.7 (Fleming et al 1996). With regard to critical appraisal, the key question to consider is whether important confounders have been identified and measured. If they have not, then the results cannot be adjusted to take account of them.

2. Is it likely that there is bias in either the selection of the cases or in the selection of the controls?

Perhaps the most difficult part of a case control study is deciding how the controls should be selected. In essence, the purpose of the controls is to provide an unbiased estimate of the prevalence of exposure in the population from which the cases are drawn. In a population-based, case control study where all cases in a defined population are identified, it is easier to select controls than in a case control study where not all cases in the population are identified. The Feeney et al study falls into the latter category, since it only included cases identified from hospital records, and not all cases from the study area. Cases managed entirely in primary care or referred to a hospital not in East Dorset would not have been included in the study. Since the cases come from a relatively ill-defined population, it is more difficult to select appropriate controls. The solution chosen by Feeney et al was to match the controls to cases by general practice, on the assumption that patients in the same practice are likely to have been referred to the same hospital.

Selection of cases can be a problem if there is the possibility of a diagnostic bias; i.e. are people more likely to be identified as cases simply because they have been exposed to the risk factor under study? For example, if general practitioners were aware that there might be an association between oral contraception and venous thromboembolism, then they might be more inclined to refer women with a swollen leg to hospital if they were taking oral contraceptives. This is unlikely to have been a major problem in Feeney et al's study, since knowledge of whether or not a person had been vaccinated against measles as a child is unlikely to have played a major part in the decision of a general practitioner to refer someone to hospital with gastrointestinal symptoms.

3. Was information on exposure obtained in a way likely to be free from bias?

Ideally, information on exposure should have been obtained in the same way for cases and controls by someone who is blinded (i.e. unaware) as to whether the individual is a case or a control. As pointed out by Montgomery et al (1997), bias might have been introduced in the study by Feeney et al since cases, but *not* controls, were approached directly for information about whether or not they had been vaccinated if their general practice and community health records were inadequate.

An example of information bias is *recall bias*, where cases may be more likely to remember exposure than controls. For example, recall bias is a problem in case control studies of congenital abnormalities, where parents of children with abnormalities may be more likely to remember exposure to possible risk factors than parents of healthy children (Swan et al 1992). Feeney et al avoided recall bias, since although they obtained exposure information from some cases directly, they relied only on documentary evidence, and not on patient memory.

What are the results? 4. What is the size of the odds ratio? 5. How large are the confidence intervals around the odds ratio?

Having decided whether or not the results are valid, the next step is to consider what they mean. There are two aspects to this: looking at the size of the odds ratio, and the size of the confidence interval around the odds ratio. The higher the odds ratio, the stronger the association between exposure and disease. The 95% confidence intervals represent the bounds within which the true odds ratio probably[2] lies given the results of the study. If the confidence intervals include 1, then no statistically significant association between exposure and disease has been observed in the study. In Feeney et al's study, the odds ratio was 0.97, with a confidence interval from 0.64 to 1.47. In other words, while no significant association was found, the results would be consistent with measles vaccination conferring a 47% increase or a 36% reduction in the risk of inflammatory bowel disease.

6. Is it likely, if an association is observed, that the relationship between exposure and disease is causal?

From a clinical point of view, one wants to be able to form a judgement as to whether or not an association between exposure and disease is causal, since this would guide whether you advised patients to avoid exposure or not. Unfortunately, case control studies cannot provide definitive proof of

---

[2] i.e. the confidence interval will contain the true value for the odds ratio 19 times out of 20 – or 95% of the time.

causality, only circumstantial evidence. In order to weigh up the likelihood that an association is causal, it is necessary to consider the evidence from a case control study in the context of other evidence that is available. A classic guideline for doing this was produced by Bradford-Hill (1965). An adaptation of this guideline is shown in Box 8.3.

Box 8.3 Is an association between exposure and disease causal?

1. *How strong is the association?*
   How large is the odds ratio (case control study), or relative risk? (cohort study)
2. *How consistent is the evidence?*
   Have different types of study in different places and at different times shown the same association between exposure and disease?
3. *Is the temporal relationship correct?*
   Does exposure precede onset of the disease?
4. *Is causation biologically plausible?*
   Does a causal link fit in with what we know already from our understanding of the basic sciences such as pathology and physiology in relation to the disease process?
5. *Is there a dose–response relationship?*
   Are people who have had greater exposure at greater risk of the disease?
6. *Is there evidence of reversibility?*
   If the risk factor is removed, does the incidence of the disease fall?
7. *Might confounding still explain the association?*
   Is it plausible that the association is due to confounding factors that have been inadequately dealt with in the studies?

---

7. How big is the risk?

Risk can be presented in two main ways: relative and absolute. An odds ratio is a relative measure of risk, in that it tells you how much more likely it is that someone who is exposed will develop the disease as compared to someone who is not exposed. It does not tell you how big the risk is for an individual, since this is dependent upon what is the individual's under-lying risk. It is not possible to derive an absolute measure of risk from a case control study without using information from other sources. For example, in the case control study of third generation oral contraceptives and risk of venous thromboembolism (Spitzer et al 1996), the odds ratio for thromboembolism in third generation users as compared to second generation users was 1.5. The authors estimated that this equated to an absolute risk of death from thromboembolism of 14 per million users per year in second generation users and 20 (approximately 1.5×14)[3] per million users per year in third generation users. They did this by finding out what the death rates for thromboembolism were from routine national statistics, and

---

[3.] It is not exactly 1.5×14 since an odds ratio is not identical to a relative risk, though it can often be thought of as being virtually equivalent to a relative risk.

assuming that the prevalence of exposure in the controls reflected the prevalence of exposure in the whole population. Thus, they could conclude that if 1 million patients were switched from third generation to second generation pills, this would prevent six deaths per year. In other words, 166 666 (million ÷ 6) women would need to switch to prevent one death. This representation of the size of the risk in absolute terms is easier to interpret when it comes to making informed choices about which pill to take.

8. Is exposure of patients in the study similar to the exposure of your own patients?

In the Feeney et al study, exposure to measles vaccine would have been during the second year of life. In some countries, however, measles vaccine is given during the first year of life. Therefore, while the study might be interpreted as reassuring for the UK, it does not necessarily provide relevant data for those countries with different vaccination programmes (Van Damme et al 1997).

STUDIES ASSESSING PROGNOSIS

As mentioned at the beginning of the chapter, observational studies, and in particular, cohort studies, can be a useful source of information about prognosis. The major criteria for assessing the validity of studies describing prognosis are shown in Box 8.4 (Laupacis et al 1994). Perhaps the most important question to consider is whether the patients in the study are representative of patients in the population as a whole. For example, studies that are based on patients who are referred to specialist centres are likely to give estimates of prognosis that are worse than studies that also include patients who are managed in primary care. This is sometimes labelled *referral filter bias*.

Box 8.4 Criteria for assessing validity of a cohort study giving information on prognosis

Key issues
1.   Was there a representative sample of patients?
2.   Were the patients at a similar point in the course of their illness?
3.   Was follow-up complete?

Secondary issues
4.   Was follow-up over a sufficient period of time?
5.   Were the outcomes used objective and unbiased?
6.   Was adjustment made for important prognostic factors?

Adapted from Laupacis et al (1994).

It also helps if the patients are at a similar point in the illness when they are entered into the study. This might be early (sometimes referred to as an *inception cohort*) or later in the course of the disease. If patients are entered into the study at different stages of an illness, then the results can be difficult to interpret since duration of illness is likely to be associated with outcome.

Completeness of follow-up is particularly important for prognosis studies, since it is likely that loss to follow-up will be associated with outcome. For example, patients who have a good outcome (i.e. remain well) may be less likely to attend follow-up, because it does not seem relevant to them. Conversely, it could be argued that patients with a poor outcome may be less likely to be followed up, either because it is too much effort for them to attend, or perhaps because they have died. Either way, the bigger the loss to follow-up, the less certain the reader can be that the prognosis observed in the patients followed up is truly representative of the prognosis in the whole study population.

CONCLUSION

Case control studies play an important role in answering questions about harm and aetiology (causation). However, because they are prone to bias, in particular as a result of confounding, the conclusions that can be drawn from any one case control study tend to be more circumspect than those that can be drawn from a well-designed, randomised controlled trial. Therefore, such articles need to be appraised carefully and interpreted in the light of whatever other evidence is available.

REFERENCES

Bradford-Hill A 1965 The environment and disease: association or causation? Journal of the Royal Society of Medicine 58:295–300
Connor R J, Prorok P C, Weed D L 1991 The case control design and the assessment of the efficacy of cancer screening. Journal of Clinical Epidemiology 44:1215–1221
Feeney M, Clegg A, Winwood P, Snook J for the East Dorset Gastroenterology Group 1997 A case-control study of measles vaccination and inflammatory bowel disease. Lancet 350:764–766
Fleming P J, Blair P S, Bacon C et al 1996 Environment of infants during sleep and risk of the sudden infant death syndrome: results of 1993–5 case control study for confidential enquiry into still births and deaths in infancy. British Medical Journal 313:191–195
Hennekens C H, Buring J E 1987 Epidemiology in medicine. Little, Brown, Boston
Jewell D P 1996 Crohn's disease. Oxford textbook of medicine, 3rd edn. Oxford University Press, Oxford, p 1936–1943
Laupacis A, Wells G, Richardson S, Tugwell P 1994 Users' guides to the medical literature. V. How to use an article about prognosis. Journal of the American Medical Association 272:234–237
Montgomery S M, Morris D L, Pounder R E, Wakefield A J 1997 Measles vaccination and inflammatory bowel disease (letter). Lancet 350:1774

Spitzer W O, Lewis M A, Heinemann L A J et al 1996 Third generation oral contraceptives and risk of venous thromboembolic disorders: an international case-control study. British Medical Journal 312:83–88

Swan S H, Shaw G M, Schulman J 1992 Reporting and selection bias in case control studies of congenital malformations. Epidemiology 3:356–363

Van Damme W, Lynen L, Kegels G, Van Lerberghe W 1997 Measles vaccination and inflammatory bowel disease (letter). Lancet 350:1774

Vessey M P, Doll R, Peto R, Johnson B, Wiggins P 1976 A long term follow up study of women using different methods of contraception – an interim report. Journal of Biosocial Sciences 8:373–427

Vessey M P, Villard-Mackintosh L, McPherson K, Yeates D 1989 Mortality among oral contraceptive users: 20 year follow up of women in a cohort study. British Medical Journal 300:330–331

9

Systematic review

Kate Seers

INTRODUCTION

Imagine it is a usual day at work. You are working with patients and you need to make a decision about the best plan of care for one particular patient. There may be one or more parts of that care where you are not sure what the best plan would be. For example, perhaps you are planning pain management, and you think that this patient might benefit from relaxation to enhance the pain relief. Is there any evidence on which to base this decision? So you start with a clinical problem; a patient with pain, and not knowing whether relaxation might help. This then is turned into a first draft of a clinical question: is relaxation effective in reducing pain? (see Ch. 2 for more details on moving from a clinical problem to a clinical question) and the clinical question is used to direct a search for evidence that can answer this question.

You may find a mountain of research papers, and it is just not feasible to read all of them. Or the amount may be more manageable, but some of the studies you find suggest the evidence is very positive, whereas others are less clear or even negative. Or perhaps there are several small studies, but you are not sure how robust their findings are. Where does that leave you with your clinical question that needs answering so that you can give the best possible care? What do you do and how do you decide what the overall evidence shows?

This chapter will look at how you try to judge studies that search for all research on a specific question and in some way combine it. If you are interested in actually undertaking such a review, then the NHS Centre for Reviews and Dissemination Report (1996) and the Cochrane Library (1998) handbook are useful resources.

One way to try to get an overview of research that might answer your clinical question is to search the literature for a systematic review of the area (see Ch. 3 for searching using 'publication type'). But what exactly is a systematic review, and how is it different from any other sort of review?

You may be familiar with the narrative reviews traditionally found in many journals. Normally someone, usually an expert, looks at the evidence in a certain area. Mulrow (1987) argues that traditional reviews do not routinely use systematic methods to identify, assess and synthesise information. Thus normally there is no methods section for the actual conduct of the review. The reader then has no way of knowing whether the review is based on a systematic review of the evidence, or on a collection of papers which the author has found in a less systematic way and thus the evidence presented may not be complete. Mulrow (1987, 1994) argues there is a need for systematic reviews of the evidence. This needs to be undertaken in just as rigorous a way as any primary piece of research, with a clear question and explicit methods for all stages of the process.

Definitions of a systematic review have identified this need to be methodical. One such definition describes a systematic review as:

a review of a clearly formulated question that uses systematic and explicit methods to identify, select and critically appraise relevant research, and to collect and analyse data from studies that are included in the review. Statistical methods may or may not be used to analyse and summarise the results of the included studies.   Cochrane Library 1998: Glossary

This should mean that another person could replicate the review, as the next definition highlights.

A systematic review is:

an attempt to minimise the element of arbitrariness ... by making explicit the review process, so that, in principle, another reviewer with access to the same resources could undertake the review and reach broadly the same conclusions.
                                                        Dixon et al (1997: 157)

Three key features of such a review are:

- a strenuous effort to locate all original reports on the topic of interest
- critical evaluation of the reports
- conclusions are drawn based on a synthesis of studies which meet preset quality criteria (Crombie & McQuay 1998: 1).

When synthesising results, a meta-analysis may be undertaken. This is: 'the use of statistical techniques in a systematic review to integrate the results of the included studies' (Cochrane Library 1998: Glossary).

A meta-analysis is thus a statistical technique for combining data (or pooling data) from several studies within a systematic review. A meta-analysis in itself does not necessarily mean the review on which it is based is systematic. The NHS Centre for Reviews and Dissemination Report (1996) suggests it may be best to pool studies on each relevant measurement of the effect of the intervention that is presented in the original studies.

WHY UNDERTAKE A SYSTEMATIC REVIEW?

There are many reasons for undertaking a systematic review, and some of these are outlined by Mulrow (1994):

- to reduce large quantities of information into smaller pieces for easier digestion

- decision-makers need to integrate critical pieces of biomedical information
- it is an efficient scientific technique
- generalisability of findings of the individual studies included can be established
- to assess consistency of relationships (e.g. same direction and same size of effect)
- explain data inconsistencies and conflicts
- increased power
- increased precision in estimates of risk or effect size
- improved reflection of reality.

Another reason for the importance of systematic reviews is outlined by Antman et al (1992). They looked at the accumulating data from randomised controlled trials (RCTs) of treatments for myocardial infarctions and the recommendations of clinical experts writing review articles and textbook chapters. They found review articles and textbooks often failed to mention important advances and in some cases potentially harmful treatments continued to be recommended by some experts.

WHERE CAN YOU FIND SYSTEMATIC REVIEWS?

Systematic reviews have been published in a variety of journals. In addition the Cochrane Collaboration provides an important resource in this area. Jadad et al (1998) found the Cochrane reviews tended to have greater methodological rigour and be updated more frequently than those published in paper-based journals. The Cochrane Collaboration is an international collaboration that is committed to 'preparing, maintaining and disseminating systematic reviews of the effects of health care' (Cochrane Collaboration 1997). It promotes and publishes the Cochrane Library. This contains the Cochrane Database of Systematic Reviews. In a recent issue (Cochrane Library 1998 issue 4) there were 481 completed reviews and protocols for an additional 438 reviews currently being undertaken. Such a review has a pre-specified protocol, where every stage of the process of undertaking the review is made explicit.

Sections covered in a protocol include background, objectives, criteria for considering studies for the review (including types of participants, types of interventions, types of outcome measure, types of study), search strategy for identification of studies, study selection, methodological quality assessment, data extraction, meta-analysis, the comparisons to be made, sub-group analysis and sensitivity analysis to be undertaken. The point to note here is that all these aspects of the protocol are set out before the review is undertaken.

Many of the systematic reviews so far completed are based on evidence of effectiveness of an intervention from RCTs. A methodology for systematic reviews using other research designs, such as observational studies, diagnosis, economic appraisal and qualitative research is much less well developed, although there are guidelines or discussions of the issues (observational studies: Egger et al 1998; diagnosis: Irwig et al 1994, Mulrow et al 1989; economics: Rigby et al 1996; and qualitative: Noblit & Hare 1988, Sandelowski et al 1997). Some Cochrane reviews in these areas are underway, for example diagnosing acute sinusitis: Varonen & Makela (1998).

CRITICAL APPRAISAL OF SYSTEMATIC REVIEWS

If you find a systematic review, how do you assess whether or not it is any good? You need to know that possible sources of bias have been minimised. One place to start is to use a guide which suggests a structured way of looking at the systematic review. One such guide has been developed by Oxman et al (1994). Other guides available include those by Dixon et al (1997) and Greenhalgh (1997).

Oxman et al (1994) break down their approach into three sections:

- Are the results valid?
- If they are, what are the results?
- Will the results help in my patient care?

Answers are, typically, yes, no or can't tell.

These three sections are further sub-divided as outlined below, with the first two questions being called a primary guide (to quickly screen out unsuitable studies) and questions 3 to 11 called secondary guides because they look at the research in more detail.

ARE THE RESULTS VALID?

Primary guides

1. Did the review address a focused clinical question? (see Ch. 2 on asking clinical questions)

If the clinical question being addressed is not clear, Oxman et al (1994) suggest moving on to the next article.

2. Were the criteria used to select articles for inclusion appropriate?

The reader needs to know what criteria were used to select the research. This should include who the study participants were, what was done and what outcomes were assessed. In addition, the methodological criteria for selecting the study should reflect the essential elements of good design in the primary study. Thus if studies included were RCTs, you would expect only studies which had randomised patients to treatments to be included. The strictness with which additional elements of good RCT design should be applied such as randomisation being adequately and appropriately described, and other criteria such as blinding or intention to treat analysis may vary, but should be explicit.

For example, if a systematic review was undertaken looking at the use of relaxation for acute pain control, studies may be restricted to randomised studies of patients aged 18 to 65 who had no pre-existing chronic pain, and had a particular type of relaxation administered in a standardised manner. Outcomes may be only changes in pain, or might be broader and include changes in anxiety, medication use or perceptions of control.

A point to consider is that the narrower the inclusion criteria, the less generalisable are the results. In the above example, it would be difficult to know how far or whether one could apply the results of such a review to patients who had chronic pain and who were over 65. Similarly, if a different type of relaxation had been used, it would be uncertain how transferable any findings might be. However, this needs to be balanced with using very broad inclusion criteria, when heterogeneity becomes an issue. Such studies may cover a wide range of patients and/or interventions and/or outcomes and the justification for then combining these differing groups comes into question.

The importance of a clear statement of inclusion criteria is that studies should be selected on the basis of these criteria (i.e. any study that matches these criteria is included) rather than selecting the study on the basis of the results.

Secondary guides

3. Is it unlikely that important relevant studies were missed?

Here you are looking for the comprehensiveness of the search. Which databases have been searched? Have any obvious ones been missed? Have the researchers checked the reference lists of articles and of textbooks, contacted experts (to get their list of references checked for completeness, tried to find out about ongoing or unpublished research) and searched for the 'grey' (unpublished) literature? Has hand-searching been used? Search terms used are also important – has an obvious MeSH term been missed or is there another term they have not used? For example, when searching for papers looking at care of the elderly, use of the term 'senior' in the North American literature may be overlooked. Are languages other than English included? This may have important implications; for example, Dickersin et al (1994) found 20% of vision trials were not in English. Unpublished data are useful to include because Egger & Davey Smith (1998) highlight how studies with significant results are more likely to be published than studies without significant results (publication bias). One way of looking for publication bias is to use a funnel plot. This is 'a graphical display of a sample size plotted against effect size for the studies included in a systematic review' (NHS Centre for Reviews and Dissemination Report 1996: 85). The points on this graph should look like a funnel, and if they do not, then some studies may not have been found or published. Egger et al (1997) have proposed a graphical test to detect bias in meta-analysis.

4. Was the validity of the included studies appraised?

Was the quality of the original studies included in the review assessed? Here you are looking to see whether the design and execution of the included studies suggest likely systematic biases.

Ensuring studies of effectiveness are randomised is important. For example, Seers & Carroll (1998) found that non-randomised studies into the effectiveness of relaxation for acute pain were much more likely to show a positive result than randomised studies. Similarly, Schultz et al (1995) found studies where randomisation was inadequately concealed could overestimate odds ratios by as much as 40%, and trials that were not double blind exaggerated odds ratios by 17%.

Whether or not one should use a quality filter to decide whether to include studies has been the subject of debate. Although Dixon et al (1997:157) argue that a systematic review 'requires ... an explicit system for grading the quality of evidence obtained', the advice from the Cochrane Library (1998: section 6.7.2) is 'None of the currently available scales for measuring the validity or 'quality' of trials can be recommended without reservation. If reviewers ... choose to use such a scale, it must be with caution.' These scales have been reviewed by Moher et al (1995), who assessed 25 scales and nine checklists. One pragmatic approach is to use some sort of quality scale, and then do a sensitivity analysis and look at the results with low quality studies in, and then with them excluded (see, for example, Sindhu 1996). This also gives an indication of the robustness of the findings of the review.

5. Were assessments of the studies reproducible?

Oxman et al (1994) point out that each decision about which studies to include, their validity and which data to extract are all subjective decisions requiring judgements which are affected by mistakes (random errors) and bias (systematic errors). They argue that having two or more people making these judgements guards against such errors. So here you are looking for more than one person reading the paper and deciding whether or not to include it.

6. Were the results similar from study to study?

In some ways this is a difficult question, because how similar is 'similar'? It is common that a variety of patients having a range of broadly similar but slightly different interventions which have been assessed using a range of outcomes are included in a systematic review. There may also be differences in study design. Is it still sensible to combine results if this is the case? One factor which may help in this decision is a test for heterogeneity. This test looks at the probability that the differences between the studies result from chance alone.

Statistical heterogeneity is when results of individual trials are to some extent incompatible with each other (Thompson 1994). It exists when there is greater variation between the results than is likely owing to chance. Thompson (1994) points out that to understand these tests, it is useful to know that the chi square statistic on which they are based has an average p value equal to its degrees of freedom. Values much larger than the degrees of freedom suggest a smaller p value and thus significant statistical heterogeneity. This means greater variation exists between the studies than is likely by chance alone. One might then conclude that the studies are so different that it makes no sense to combine them.

Since this test of heterogeneity is described as having a low power (Thompson 1994), a non-significant test cannot be interpreted as evidence of homogeneity. Thompson suggests that the guiding principle should be to investigate the influences of specific clinical differences between the studies, rather than relying on an overall statistical test of heterogeneity. Clinical and statistical heterogeneity need to be distinguished. Clinical heterogeneity refers to differences between settings, patients, techniques and outcomes, which might lead you to suggest it does not make sense to combine the data.

WHAT ARE THE RESULTS?

7. What do the results of a systematic review mean?

Terms that you will probably come across when looking at systematic reviews include vote counting, odds ratios, relative risks, weighted mean differences and fixed and random effects.

Vote counting. If a systematic review does not contain a meta-analysis, the results may be presented as a simple vote count, that is, the number of studies supporting, for example, an intervention and the number not supporting it. Problems associated with vote counting need to be kept in mind when interpreting these results, such as equal weight being given to each study, regardless of size.

Binary or continuous data. The type of data will dictate what you see when you look at a meta-analysis.

1. Binary data (e.g. an event rate: something that happens or it does not – myocardial infarction, stroke, improved/not improved) is usually combined using odds ratios. (Methods exist for combining relative risks

and risk differences. Note that absolute risk reduction and risk differences are synonomous.) Numbers needed to treat (NNTs) can also be helpful here (see Ch. 14 on therapy for more details on NNTs) and McQuay & Moore (1997) argue for systematic reviews to produce an NNT so that results from systematic reviews can be more easily applied in practice.

2. Continuous data (e.g. numbers of days, peak expiratory flow rate) are combined using differences in mean values for treatment and control groups (weighted mean differences or WMD) when units of measurement are the same (e.g. all using the same anxiety scale), or standardised mean differences when units of measurement differ (e.g. using a variety of anxiety scales, where one numerical value could mean very different things, depending on the scale used). Here the difference in means is divided by the pooled standard deviation.

Thus when you look at a meta-analysis, you will see odds ratios and/or weighted mean differences or standardised mean differences, depending on the outcomes measures that have been used in the included studies.

Odds ratio.   What are the odds and where does the ratio come into it? The odds look at how much a treatment affects an event rate. The odds of an event are the probability of it occurring compared to the probability of it not occurring. The odds ratio is the ratio of the odds of an event in the treatment (or exposed) group compared to the odds in the control (or unexposed) group (see Ch. 8). Relative risk and absolute risk reduction may also be used to express these sorts of differences between a treatment and control group.

Relative risk   (also known as risk ratio). 'The risk (proportion, probability or rate) is the ratio of people with an event compared to the total in that group' (Cochrane Library 1998). A relative risk is the risk in the treatment group compared to the risk in the control group. A relative risk of 1 means there is no difference between the groups (see Ch. 14 to see how the calculation of relative risks differs from odds ratios).

Relative risk is appealing because it is easier to understand than the rather abstract notion (to non-gamblers at least!) of an odds. There is debate over whether relative risks should be used in preference to odds ratios (see Deeks 1996), but odds ratios are commonly used. In case control studies relative risks cannot be calculated (because the disease prevalence is not known), so odds ratios are used. If an event is rare, odds ratios and relative risks will be similar. Around a 10 to 20% event rate they start becoming different and if an event is common, they can be very different with the odds ratio showing a larger effect than the relative risk.

What do these odds and relative risks mean in plain English? Let's say a study looked at the odds of getting inadequate pain relief with relaxation compared to the odds of getting inadequate pain relief without relaxation. If the odds ratio was 0.70, this would mean you had 30% reduction in the odds of having inadequate pain relief with relaxation, compared to without relaxation. If the relative risk was 0.82, this would mean patients' risk of having inadequate pain relief is 18% less if they had relaxation.

What do odds ratios used in a meta-analysis look like?   See Figure 9.1. The square box or 'blob' on the figure (which is sometimes known colloquially as a 'blobogram') is the individual study effect (technically referred to as the point estimate) with its associated confidence intervals as lines either side of that box (technically known as the interval estimate). Sometimes the size of the box may vary to reflect the weight that particular study is given, with larger boxes representing higher weighting. Lower weighted studies are usually those with smaller samples and large confidence intervals. The overall or summary effect (from combining or pooling the studies) is usually depicted as a diamond. Lau et al (1998) argue that since patients may respond differently to treatment, this pooling may need to be supplanted by summarising evidence along multiple covariates of interest. They conclude that 'patients' heterogeneity should be anticipated and sought up front, not ignored in pursuit of aggregate statistical significance' (Lau et al 1998: 127). Thus, although one overall number is appealing in its simplicity, it may oversimplify a more complex situation.

An odds ratio of 1 on a linear scale means there is no difference between the experimental and control group. This value of 1 is the line down the middle of the figure (sometimes with the wording 'favours treatment' on one side and 'favours control' on the other). If the confidence interval does **not** cross the line, it means that there is a 95% chance that there is a true difference between the groups. That is, that there is a significant difference on that particular outcome between the intervention and control groups.

Whether this favours the treatment or control will depend on which side of the vertical line the confidence interval appears. The left-hand side is less of something, and the right-hand side is more of something. Whether this is 'good' or 'bad' depends on the variable. For example, fewer years alive might be 'bad' if you are aiming to improve survival, whereas fewer heart attacks might be 'good' if this was your intent. If the confidence interval does cross this vertical line labelled '1', it means that any difference in that outcome between the treatments could have occurred by chance (i.e. there are no significant differences, equal odds are plausible, there is no treatment effect). It may be that a very wide confidence interval is due to a very small sample size, and it would reduce with more people in the study. A 95% confidence interval covers likely results from a set of similar studies. It therefore provides a more realistic view of what will happen in practice than a point estimate, because it takes potential variability into account.

It is worth noting that a lack of evidence for an intervention is not the same as evidence of a lack of effect.

Odds ratios are usually plotted on a log scale. This is because if we assume a desirable or good outcome of a particular treatment meant you had less of something (such as fewer strokes or fewer anxiety attacks), on a linear

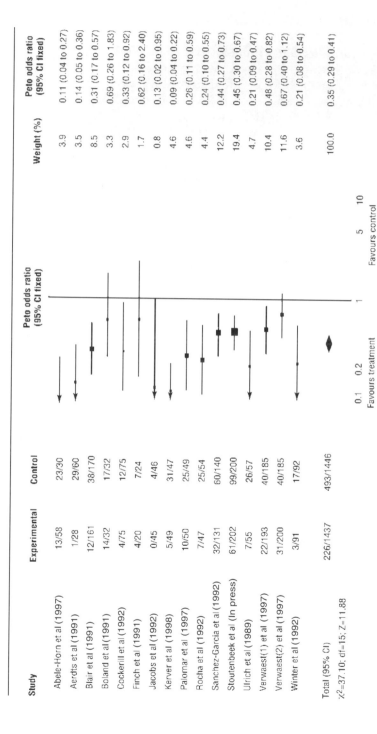

Study	Experimental	Control	Peto odds ratio (95% CI fixed)	Weight (%)	Peto odds ratio (95% CI fixed)
Abele-Horn et al (1997)	13/58	23/30		3.9	0.11 (0.04 to 0.27)
Aerdts et al (1991)	1/28	29/60		3.5	0.14 (0.05 to 0.36)
Blair et al (1991)	12/161	38/170		8.5	0.31 (0.17 to 0.57)
Boland et al (1991)	14/32	17/32		3.3	0.69 (0.26 to 1.83)
Cockerill et al (1992)	4/75	12/75		2.9	0.33 (0.12 to 0.92)
Finch et al (1991)	4/20	7/24		1.7	0.62 (0.16 to 2.40)
Jacobs et al (1992)	0/45	4/46		0.8	0.13 (0.02 to 0.95)
Kerver et al (1998)	5/49	31/47		4.6	0.09 (0.04 to 0.22)
Palomar et al (1997)	10/50	25/49		4.6	0.26 (0.11 to 0.59)
Rocha et al (1992)	7/47	25/54		4.4	0.24 (0.10 to 0.55)
Sanchez-Garcia et al (1992)	32/131	60/140		12.2	0.44 (0.27 to 0.73)
Stoutenbeek et al (In press)	61/202	99/200		19.4	0.45 (0.30 to 0.67)
Ulrich et al (1989)	7/55	26/57		4.7	0.21 (0.09 to 0.47)
Verwaest(1) et al (1997)	22/193	40/185		10.4	0.48 (0.28 to 0.82)
Verwaest(2) et al (1997)	31/200	40/185		11.6	0.67 (0.40 to 1.12)
Winter et al (1992)	3/91	17/92		3.6	0.21 (0.08 to 0.54)
Total (95% CI)	226/1437	493/1446		100.0	0.35 (0.29 to 0.41)

$\chi^2 = 37.10$; df = 15; Z = 11.88

0.1   0.2   1   5   10

Favours treatment   Favours control

Figure 9.1   Meta-analysis of the effect of combined topical and systemic antibiotics as prophylaxis for respiratory tract infections in patients in intensive care units. This figure illustrates the different weights given to different studies (the different sized square boxes) and the overall effect (the diamond). The figure shows there is a strong protective effect of combined topical and systemic antibiotics in this group of patients, with an overall effect odds ratio of 0.35 (CI 0.29–0.41). Thus patients having this combination reduced their incidence of respiratory tract infection by 65%. This figure was first published in the BMJ: D'Amico R, Pifferi S, Leonetti C, Torri V, Tinazzi A, Liberati A 1998 Effect of antibiotic prophylaxis in critically ill adult patients: a systematic review of randomised controlled trials. British Medical Journal 316:1275–1285 and is reproduced by permission of the BMJ).

scale 0 to 1 would equal 'good', whereas 1 to infinity would equal 'bad'. This is clearly visually unbalanced and using a log scale gives an equal line length for good and bad. If odds ratios are plotted on a log scale, then a log odds ratio of 0 means no effect and whether or not the 95% confidence interval crosses a vertical line through zero will lead to a decision about its significance.

The other terms that are often seen in meta-analysis include the type of model used.

Fixed effects model. This ignores between-study heterogeneity and estimates treatment effect as if it were a single true value underlying all study results. That is, it assumes the treatment effect in all studies is the same and it ignores between-study variability. Any differences are described as the result of random (sampling) error within studies.

For binary data, tests used include Mantel–Haenszel method and the Peto method.

For continuous data, tests used include the weighted mean of study effects (if measures are on the same scale), or standardised mean effect sizes, or 'd-statistics' (if measures are on different scales).

Random effects model. This assumes individual study effect sizes will exhibit random variation, as they are a random sample from a population of effect sizes (Sindhu 1998). Differences between studies are thus a combination of random (sampling) error and variation between studies. This estimate is likely to be more conservative with a wider confidence interval. The NHS Centre for Reviews and Dissemination Report (1996) suggests both are reported. Tests used in random effects are known as the DerSimonian–Laird method (DerSimonian & Laird 1986).

Diagnostic tests. Here you do not have an odds ratio. You will be looking at sensitivity/specificity, positive/negative predictive values or likelihood ratios.

Receiver-operating characteristic (ROC) curves mean several studies can be displayed (see Ch. 13 on diagnosis). The plot can show how differences in cut-off points taken can affect, for example, sensitivity and specificity, or true positive and false positive rates. The top left-hand corner represents maximum joint specificity and sensitivity or maximum true positive rate and minimum false positive rates.

Meta-regression. This is relatively new in meta-analysis. Lau et al (1998:124) describe it as an 'attempt to identify significant relations between the treatment effect … and the covariates of interest.' The unit of observation is the study or sub-group, rather than the individual patient. Lau et al (1998) argue that it may provide more insight than traditional pooling, as data can be modelled along one or multiple dimensions.

8. How precise are the results?

This is asking whether there are any confidence intervals used, so the reader can see the range of values around the effect size, where one is 95%

confident that the 'true' effect would lie. The Cochrane Library (1998), section 6.1, defines precision as 'a measure of the likelihood of random errors. It is reflected in the confidence interval around the estimate of effect from each study ... more precise results are given more weight.' Thus the more precise the results, the narrower (smaller) the confidence interval. For example, an odds ratio of 0.35 and 95% confidence interval 0.22–0.56 shows the confidence interval does not cross the line (the value of 1) and there is a significant difference between the groups; an odds ratio of 1.12 and 95% confidence interval 0.75–1.67 clearly does cross the line (the value of 1) and the difference between groups is not significant.

WILL THE RESULTS HELP ME IN CARING FOR MY PATIENTS?

9. Can the results be applied to my patient care?

How similar are the patients you care for to those included in the review? The wider the type of patients included in the review, the more likely you are to feel the results may apply across a range of different patients. However, it is sometimes a difficult decision to know whether, for example, something that works on men will be equally effective with women, or something that works in younger people will work in the same way in older people.

Sub-group analysis may be one way of addressing this concern, although there are concerns with this approach (e.g. Counsell et al 1994, Oxman & Guyatt 1992), especially if the study is not powered to consider sub-groups, and the sub-groups are not specified before the study starts. Sub-group analysis may be more like a fishing trip (to try to find significant results) when, in fact, the play of chance may have more to do with apparently significant results than any intrinsic differential effect of the intervention, as the Counsell et al (1994) article clearly highlighted. They looked at sub-group analysis and concluded that chance influences the outcome of clinical trials and systematic reviews much more than many investigators realise and this may lead to incorrect conclusions about the benefit of treatment. Davey Smith et al (1997) argue that you often need individual patient data for meaningful sub-group analysis. Clarke & Stewart (1997) similarly argue for the use of individual patient data to improve the reliability of meta-analysis, but also highlight the difficulties of obtaining such data.

10. Were all clinically important outcomes considered?

What is clinically important can depend on your perspective. Sometimes whilst factors like bone density may be included in a review to assess the effectiveness of certain orthopaedic procedures, it may be some other outcome, like the ability to get to the shops, that needs to be considered and this sort of outcome may be crucial from the patient's perspective.

11. Are the benefits worth the harms and costs?

This may cover a range of factors, like benefit of early treatment following a positive cervical smear versus the harms of high anxiety. Or it may be the benefits of a chemotherapeutic agent versus its unpleasant side effects. An economic evaluation may be included (see Ch. 10).

These criteria suggested by Oxman et al (1994) are worth considering when critically appraising a systematic review. But they can also create difficulties. When you use a set of criteria like this, you may end up with a variety of 'no's' or 'can't tell's' in answer to the questions you pose. It is sometimes difficult to decide when a review is 'too bad' to give you any confidence in the findings. Perhaps one pragmatic approach would be that when you have several 'no's' or 'can't tell's' you are more wary about the validity and robustness of the review's findings. What this does illustrate is that, like undertaking a systematic review, critically appraising these reviews is not an exact science, but there are many subjective decisions along the way. Just like undertaking a systematic review, making explicit your decisions in the critical appraisal is therefore very important.

It may be useful to ponder that although a systematic review can provide you with high quality evidence, clinical experience and patient preferences are an important part of evidence-based health care (Sackett et al 1997). It may be that even high quality evidence does not apply to a particular patient. Similarly, Cochrane reviews do not include recommendations, as reviewers cannot know the local situation or the patient, and this is the province of the health professional caring for the patient.

LIMITATIONS OF SYSTEMATIC REVIEWS AND META-ANALYSIS

Crombie & McQuay (1998) point out that it is important not to overstate potential limitations, as systematic reviews are a major advance on both the traditional review and the use of selected evidence that went before. However, there are some limitations. Crombie & McQuay (1998) raise the possibility that sometimes a review may mislead. They argue this can occur when the quality of the review is poor or when publication bias occurs. Thus a review may overestimate the effectiveness of the treatment/intervention. If the results of a review (which may combine several small trials) are compared to those of a large RCT, the results may not be the same. For example, Cappelleri et al (1996) found over 80% of 79 reviews agreed with large trials. LeLorier et al (1997) found a 65% agreement, although this article has been criticised by Naylor & Davey Smith (1998).

Eysenck (1995) argues that meta-analysis is often used to recover something from poor studies. He also argues against combining varied treatments and end points.

Meta-analysis may be seen as concerned with the whole population, rather than an individual patient. However, with the shift away from a summary statistic to looking at multiple covariates that Lau et al (1998) advocate, their goal for meta-analysis of 'knowing how best to treat the individual' perhaps comes a little closer.

Acknowledgement

Many thanks to Nicola Crichton for her helpful comments on drafts of this chapter.

REFERENCES

Abele-Horn M, Dauber A, Bauernfeind A et al 1997 Decrease in nosocomial pneumonia ventilated patients by selective oropharyngeal decontamination (SPO). Intensive Care Medicine 23:187–195.
Aerdts S J A, van Dalen R, Clasener H A L, Festen J, van Lier H J J, Vollaard E J 1991 Antibiotic prophylaxis of respiratory tract infection in mechanically ventilated patients. Chest 100:783–791
Antman E M, Lau J, Kupelnick B, Mosteller F, Chalmers T C 1992 A comparison of the results of meta-analyses of randomised controlled trials and recommendations of clinical experts. Treatments for myocardial infarction. Journal of the American Medical Association 268 (2):240–248
Blair P, Rowlands B J, Lowry K, Webb H, Amstrong P, Smilie J 1991 Selective decontamination of the digestive tract: a stratified, randomized, prospective study in a mixed intensive care unit. Surgery 110:303–310
Boland J P, Sadler D L, Stewart W, Wood D J, Zerick W, Snodgrass K R 1991 Reduction of nosocomial respiratory tract infections in the multiple trauma patients requiring mechanical ventilation by selective parenteral and enteral antisepsis regimen (SPEAR) in the intensive care [abstract]. Seventeenth congress of chemotherapy, Berlin, No 0465
Cappelleri J C, Ionnidis J P A, Schmid C H, deFerrfanti S D, Aubert M, Chalmers T C, Lau J 1996 Large trials vs meta-analysis of smaller trials: how do their results compare? Journal of the American Medical Association 276:1332–1338
Chalmers I, Altman D (eds) 1995 Systematic reviews. British Medical Journal Publishing Group, London
Clarke M J, Stewart L A 1997 Meta-analyses using individual patient data. Journal of Evaluation in Clinical Practice 3 (3):207–212
Cochrane Collaboration 1997 The Cochrane Collaboration, Oxford.
Cochrane Library 1998 Issues 2,3 & 4. Update Software, London
Cockerill F R III, Muller S R, Anhalt J P et al 1992 Prevention of infection in critically ill patients by selective decontamination of the digestive tract. Annals of Internal Medicine 117:545–553
Counsell C E, Clarke M J, Slattery J, Sandercock P A G 1994 The miracle of DICE therapy for acute stroke: fact or fictional product of sub group analysis. British Medical Journal 309:1677–1681
Crombie I K, McQuay H 1998 The systematic review: a good guide rather than guarantee. Pain 76:1–2
Davey Smith G, Egger M, Phillips A N 1997 Beyond the grand mean? British Medical Journal 315:1610–1614
Deeks J 1996 Swots corner: What is an odds ratio? Bandolier 3(issue 25):6–7
DerSimonian R, Laird N 1986 Meta-analysis in clinical trials. Controlled Clinical Trials 7:177–188

Dickersin K, Scherer R, Lefebvre C 1994 Identifying relevant studies for systematic reviews. British Medical Journal 309:1286–1291

Dixon R A, Munro J F, Silcocks P B 1997 The evidence based medicine workbook. Critical appraisal for clinical problem solving. Butterworth–Heinemann, Oxford

Egger M, Davey Smith G 1998 Bias in location and selection of studies. British Medical Journal 316:61–66

Egger M, Schneider M, Davey Smith G 1998 Meta-analysis. Spurious precision? Meta-analysis of observational studies. British Medical Journal 316:140–144

Egger M, Davey Smith G, Schneider M, Minder C 1997 Bias in meta-analysis detected by a simple graphical test. British Medical Journal 315:629–634

Eysenck H J 1995 Problems with meta-analysis. In: Chalmers I, Altman D G (eds) Systematic reviews. British Medical Journal Publishing London, ch. 6, p 64–74

Finch R G, Tomlinson P, Holliday M, Sole K, Stack C, Rocker G 1991 Selective decontamination of the digestive tract (SDD) in the prevention of secondary sepsis in a medical/surgical intensive care unit [abstract]. Seventeenth international congress of chemotherapy. Berlin, No 0471

Greenhalgh T 1997 How to read a paper. The basics of evidence based medicine. British Medical Journal Publishing, London

Irwig L, Tosteson A N A, Gatsonis C, Lau J, Colditz G, Chalmers T C, Mosteller F 1994 Guidelines for meta-analyses: evaluating diagnostic tests. Annals of Internal Medicine 120 (8):667–676

Jacobs S. Foweraker JE, Roberts SE 1992 Effectiveness of selective decontamination of the digestive tract (SDD) in an ICU with a policy encouraging a low gastric pH. Clin Intensive Medicine 3:52–58

Jadad A R, Cook D J, Jones A, Klassen T P, Tugwell P, Moher M, Moher D 1998 Methodology and reports of systematic reviews and meta-analyses. Journal of the American Medical Association 280 (3):278–280

Kerver A J H, Rommes J H, Mevissen-Verhage E A E et al 1988 Prevention of colonization and infection in critically ill patients: a prospective randomized study. Critical Care Medicine 16:1087

Lau J, Ioannidis J P A, Schmid C H 1998 Summing up evidence: one answer is not always enough. Lancet 351:123–127

LeLorier J, Georgoire G, Benhaddad A, Lapierre J, Derderian F 1997 Discrepancies between meta-analysis and subsequent large randomised controlled trials. New England Journal of Medicine 337:536–542

Lenhart F P, Unertl K, Neeser G, Ruckdeschel G, Eckart J, Peter K 1994 Selective decontamination (SDD) and sucralfate for prevention of acquired infections in intensive care [abstract]. Seventeenth international congress chemotherapy, Vienna, K101

McQuay H J, Moore R A 1997 Using numerical results from systematic reviews in clinical practice. Annals of Internal Medicine 126 (9):712–720

Moher D, Jadad A R, Nichol G, Penman M, Tugwell P, Walsh S 1995 Assessing quality of randomised controlled trials: an annotated bibliography of scales and checklists. Controlled Clinical Trials 16:62–73

Mulrow C D 1987 The medical review article: state of the science. Annals of Internal Medicine 106:485–488

Mulrow C 1994 Rationale for systematic reviews. British Medical Journal 309:597–599

Mulrow C D, Linn W D, Gaul M K, Pugh J A 1989 Assessing the quality of a diagnostic test evaluation. Journal of General Internal Medicine 4:288–294

NHS Centre for Reviews and Dissemination 1996 Undertaking systematic reviews of research on effectiveness. CRD guidelines for those carrying out or commissioning reviews. CRD Report 4. NHS CRD, University of York, York

Naylor C D, Davey Smith G 1998 Test meta-analyses for stability (Letter). British Medical Journal 317:206

Noblit G W, Hare R D 1988 Meta-ethnography: synthesising qualitative studies. Sage, Newbury Park

Oxman A D, Cook D J, Guyatt G H 1994 Users' guides to the medical literature. VI. How to use an overview. Journal of the American Medical Association 272 (17):1367–1371

Oxman A D, Guyatt G H 1992 A consumer's guide to subgroup analysis. Annals of Internal Medicine 116:78–84

Palomar M, Alvarez-Lerma F, Jorda R, Bermejo B, for the Catalan Study Group of Nosocomial Pneumonia Prevention 1997 Prevention of nosocomial infection in mechanically ventilated patients: selective digestive decontamination versus sucralfate. Clin Intensive Care 8:228–235

Rigby K, Silagy C, Crockett A 1996 Health economic reviews – are they compiled systematically? International Journal of Technology Assessment in Health Care 12 (3):450–459

Rocha L A, Martin M J, Pita S et al 1992 Prevention of nosocomial infection in critically ill patients by selective decontamination of digestive tract. Intensive Care Medicine 18:398–404

Sackett D L, Richardson W S, Rosenberg W, Haynes R B 1997 Evidence based medicine. How to practise and teach EBM. Churchill Livingstone, Edinburgh

Sanchez-Garcia M, Cambronero J A, Lopez J et al 1992 Reduced incidence of nosocomial pneumonia and shorter ICU stay in intubated patients with the use of selective decontamination of the digestive tract (SDD). A multicentric, double blind, placebo-controlled study [abstract]. European Congress on Intensive Care Medicine. Barcelona, No 0391

Sandelowski M, Docherty S, Emden C 1997 Qualitative metasynthesis: issues and techniques. Research in Nursing and Health 20:365–371

Schultz K F, Chalmers I, Hayes R J, Altman D G 1995 Empirical evidence of bias. Dimensions of methodological quality associated with estimates of treatment effects in controlled trials. Journal of the American Medical Association 273 (5):408–412

Seers K, Carroll D 1998 Relaxation techniques for acute pain management: a systematic review. Journal of Advanced Nursing 27:466–475

Sindhu F 1996 Are non-pharmacological nursing interventions for the management of pain effective? – A meta-analysis. Journal of Advanced Nursing 24:1152–1159

Sindhu F 1998 Meta-analyses and systematic reviews of the literature. In: Roe B, Webb C (eds) Research and development in clinical nursing practice. Whurr, London, ch 6, p 84–111

Stoutenbeck C P, Van Saene H K F, Little R A, Whitehead A (in press) The effect of selective decontamination of the digestive tract on mortality in multiple trauma patients. Annals of Surgery

Thompson S G 1994 Why sources of heterogeneity in meta-analysis should be investigated. British Medical Journal 309:1351–1355

Ulrich C, Harinck-deWeerd JE, Bakker NC, Jacz K, Doornbos L, de Ridder VA 1989 Selective decontamination of the digestive tract with norfloxacin in the prevention of ICU-acquired infections: a prospective randomized study. Intensive Care Medicine 15:424–431

Varonen H, Makela M 1998 Ultrasonography, radiography and clinical examination in the diagnosis of acute maxillary sinusitis in primary health care. (Cochrane review). In: The Cochrane library, Issue 2. Update Software, Oxford

Verwaest C, Verhaegen J, Ferdinande P et al 1997 Randomized, controlled trial of selective digestive decontamination in 600 mechanically ventilated patients in a multidisciplinary intensive care unit. Critical Care Medicine 25:63–71

Winter R, Humphreys H, Pick A, MacGowan A P, Willatts S M, Speller D C E 1992 A controlled trial of selective decontamination of the digestive tract in intensive care and its effect on nosocomial infection. Journal of Antimicrobial Chemotherapy 30:73–87

10

Economic evaluation

Alastair Gray

INTRODUCTION

Economic evaluation is a burgeoning part of health technology assessment, and the methodology of economic evaluation is rapidly evolving. Although what constitutes good practice is by no means written in stone, it seems clear that many economic evaluations published in the recent past have not adhered to basic principles. For example, one study (Udvarhelyi et al 1992) looked at 77 cost-effectiveness and cost-benefit articles published during the periods 1978 to 1980 and 1985 to 1987. In the articles assessed, they found in relation to six fundamental principles of analysis that just three out of the 77 adhered to all six principles. The median number of principles adhered to was three, and there was no evidence of improvement in performance over time. Similar results have been obtained from other reviews (Gerard 1992). Partly as a result of such studies, there has been a major effort amongst health economists to reach consensus on what principles should and should not be used, and clear guidelines on good practice now exist for the conduct of studies, for the preparation of manuscripts, and for journal referees and editors assessing submissions (CCOHTA 1997; Drummond et al 1997; Gold et al 1996).

In Chapter 15 we will look in detail at the cost-effectiveness approach, and ask how the results of such studies can be used in evidence-based practice. But first it is necessary to establish some basic principles. Here, we set out a checklist condensed from the conclusions of the Panel on Cost-Effectiveness in Health and Medicine, which was convened at the instigation of the US Public Health Service to produce an explicit set of guidelines for the conduct of cost-effectiveness analyses (Gold et al 1996).

A. THE FRAMEWORK

1. The type of analysis being performed should be clearly stated and justified.

Economic evaluation consists of a small family of analyses, which are conceptually distinct as can be seen from Figure 10.1. The most elementary type of study is a *cost analysis*, in which there is no information on outcomes, or possibly where there is not even any attempt to compare alternative courses

---

BOX 10.1   Checklist adapted from Gold et al (1996)

A. The framework
1. The type of analysis being performed should be clearly stated and justified.
2. The background of the problem being addressed, and the general design of the programme under investigation, including the target population, should be stated.
3. The comparator programme should be described.
4. The perspective and time horizon of the study should be stated.

B. Data and methods
5. All resources of interest in the analysis should be clearly identified, measured and valued.
6. All outcomes of interest in the analysis should be clearly identified, measured and valued.
7. Methods of obtaining estimates of effectiveness, resource use, unit costs and quality-of-life valuations should be given, alongside the sources of information.

C. Results
8. The base case results in terms of costs, effectiveness, and incremental cost-effectiveness ratios, and the uncertainty surrounding them, should be clearly set out.
9. The results should be placed in the context of other relevant economic evaluations.

D. Discussion
10. The relevance of the study for policy questions, and any ethical or distributive implications, should be discussed.

---

of action. The usefulness of this type of study is limited, as it gives no information on health outcome consequences. If there is information on the outcome or effectiveness of two alternatives, and they are known to be equivalent, then the main interest is in identifying and choosing the least cost option, and this is called a *cost-minimisation study*. However, if the outcome is known to be different, then we are in the realm of *cost-effectiveness analysis*. Here, we are interested in the difference in costs between a programme and a specified alternative, as a ratio of the difference in outcomes. Examples might include the cost per case detected of population screening compared with opportunistic screening; or the cost per life saved or life-year gained of thrombolytic therapy following myocardial infarction. In some circumstances, the outcome may best be measured in quality-adjusted life-years (QALYs), a composite measure of changes in survival and quality of life. Cost-effectiveness analyses which make use of QALYs as the principal outcome measure are sometimes called *cost–utility analyses*, the reason being that economists are interested in measuring the value or utility derived from a state of health or health change.

Note that cost-effectiveness and cost–utility analyses are premised on the assumption that the outcome – lives saved, cases detected – is worth attaining. The only question they address is 'Given that this is a worthwhile objective, what is the most efficient way of attaining it?' But some studies (a small number at present) attempt to ask a more fundamental question: is

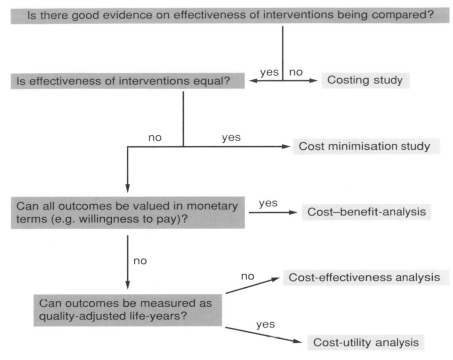

Figure 10.1   Types of economic evaluation.

the objective worth pursuing at all? For example, if it were possible in some way to place a monetary value on a life, then any action or intervention which saved a life for less than that value – that is, where the costs were less than the benefits – would be worthwhile, while any action which costs more than that value – where the costs were greater than the benefits – would not be worthwhile. This is *cost–benefit analysis*; it has the advantage of a very straightforward decision-rule, but the disadvantage that getting agreement on monetary valuations of outcomes is very difficult.

2. The background of the problem being addressed, and the general design of the programme under investigation, including the target population, should be stated.

This is a simple but important point that many published studies unfortunately fail to comply with. Unless the background is clearly stated and the programme design and target population are clearly specified, it will be difficult to draw conclusions about the relevance of the results. Relevant aspects of the programme may include the specific technology employed, the grade and experience of staff delivering the intervention, and the physical setting, all of which may affect the costs and outcomes reported. Relevant aspects of the target population to note include their age, sex, and ethnic composition, and their baseline risk characteristics.

3. The comparator programme should be described.

As noted above, economic evaluation is concerned with comparing an intervention with some alternative. Consequently the comparator that is selected is crucial to the results. If the cost-effectiveness of a new anti-hypertensive drug was to be calculated against the alternative of no treatment, it would undoubtedly appear as much more cost-effective than if compared with existing practice, which probably includes lifestyle advice and beta-blockers. So the status quo, or current practice, will usually be the appropriate comparator.

4. The perspective and time horizon of the study should be stated.

Suppose a health authority is trying to decide whether to introduce 'a hospital at home' scheme to encourage earlier discharge from medical wards. It may save hospital resources but increase primary care costs. It may mean additional informal care from families and friends, but lead to earlier recovery and a more rapid return to paid employment. Which perspective should we adopt? The health service view alone, or the impact on informal carers, or the broad impact across society as a whole? The health service decision-maker may only be interested in health care resources, and may wish to discharge patients from hospital as rapidly as possible. But from a societal point of view it would be wise to consider these wider costs, and indeed if they are completely ignored, the treatment may be unacceptable to patients.

An illustration of this is given in Table 10.1, which is adapted from a study of the likely economic consequences of introducing varicella (chickenpox) vaccination in the USA (Lieu et al 1994). With no vaccination programme, the health care system incurs annual costs of $90m, and parents incur annual costs of $439m, mainly as a result of taking time off work to look after sick children being kept off school. If a vaccination programme were introduced, the vaccination programme itself ($88m per annum) and the residual disease costs of $10m (the vaccine being not completely effective) would fall on the health care system, so that from its perspective the annual costs would actually rise from $90m to $98m each year. However, the costs to parents would fall dramatically – from $439m to $48m each year – and society as a whole will benefit as parents' savings far outweigh the additional health care costs. So should the programme go ahead? The point is that it all depends on the perspective you adopt, but it is good practice in economic evaluations to adopt the widest perspective possible, especially if there is reason to think that different perspectives may alter the result.

Table 10.1 The importance of the perspective adopted: the example of varicella-related costs with and without a projected US vaccination programme for children ($US million 1990)

	No vaccination	Vaccination	Net cost (savings) of vaccination vs no vaccination
Medical costs vaccine and administration	0	88	88
Varicella disease costs	90	10	(80)
Total medical costs	90	98	8
Work-loss costs (savings)	439	48	(392)
Total medical + work-loss varicella-related costs (savings)	**529**	**146**	**(384)**

The time horizon of a study should extend sufficiently far into the future to capture the main economic consequences and health outcomes. This may in practice mean that a patient's full lifetime is the appropriate horizon. For example, suppose that a trial has demonstrated that a new drug is more effective than existing therapies at lowering cholesterol over a 1-year period. An economist would almost certainly want to consider the health outcomes of this change in terms of lower risk of fatal and non-fatal coronary events, and the longer term cost consequences of continuing drug therapy but also fewer coronary events. This would probably extend over a lifetime, and consequently some modelling – for example, statistically extrapolating these effects into the future – would be required.

A final point to be made about the time horizon concerns *discounting*. The costs and health outcomes of a programme or service are usually spread over time, and may differ widely between programmes. For instance, the direct costs of influenza immunisation are incurred immediately, and the benefits (in terms of health effects and treatment costs avoided) are also attained more or less immediately; in contrast, the costs of a school anti-smoking health education campaign are incurred immediately, but the benefits will be attained a long time into the future. To compare these programmes at a point in time – the present – it is necessary to place the stream of future costs on a common basis of present values, by adjusting future costs and outcomes using a discount rate so that they are given less weight than present costs and outcomes.

There are two main reasons for discounting. The first is *time preference*: generally we prefer to receive benefits now rather than in the future, and to postpone costs to the future rather than bear them now. We value present benefits more highly than future benefits, and perceive present costs to be higher than future costs. The second concerns *opportunity cost* again: resources not spent now could be invested at a real rate of return, and would be worth more in real terms in the future. If the real rate of return is 5% per annum, then £100 invested now would equal £128 in 5 years, and conversely £100 in 5 years would equal £77 now. So if you knew that you would need £100 in 5 years, you could invest £77. This is the basis of pension plans. Put another way, if you were owed £100 and were offered the choice of having it now or in 5 years' time, what would you choose? (The actual discount rate used has been the subject of some debate, and varies between countries. At present in the UK the standard discount rate for costs and outcomes in economic evaluations is 6% per annum, but it would be considered good practice to display results using a range of different discount rates, including zero.)

B. DATA AND METHODS
5. All resources of interest in the analysis should be clearly identified, measured and valued.

Estimating the costs of an intervention is usually done in distinct stages. First, it is necessary to identify all the resources involved in the intervention itself and any future resource consequences such as adverse events or an altered probability of clinical events (hence the need for a clear description of the intervention). For example, the resource consequences of hormone replacement therapy include not only the drug therapy itself but also an altered future likelihood of osteoporosis, breast cancer, endometrial cancer and possibly cardiovascular and other diseases, all of which have resource consequences. Ideally we should include not only health care resources, but also the consequences for patients, their families and society (see the discussion of the study perspective above).

Second, after these resource consequences have been identified, they need to be measured and then valued. The way in which they are measured will vary depending on the level of detail of the study. For example, use of hospital resources may be measured simply in terms of numbers of cases or of in-patient days, or in much more detail by documenting all the nursing and medical time, drugs and dressings, tests and consumables involved in the episode. The level of detail in turn will depend on the research question: is there reason to believe that the intensity of care in hospital may differ between interventions, for example, or is it more important simply to detect any overall difference in hospitalisation rates?

The valuation of these resources is the point at which unit costs are attached. To an economist, cost is measured in terms of the potential opportunities which are foregone when resources are committed to one purpose rather than another. The normal market price – the wage for a nurse or the price of a prescribed drug – will usually be a reasonable measure of this opportunity cost. However, prices, charges, tariffs or fees can sometimes be misleading. For example, a family planning clinic may get 'free' space in a hospital out-patient department: that is, it does not pay for it. But by using the space in this way, other potential benefits from using the space in a different way are sacrificed. So there is an opportunity cost, even though there is no charge. This distinction can become very important in areas such as informal care, where relatives and friends of patients may be sacrificing a great deal of work time or leisure time to caring, for no financial reward. There is no price, but the opportunity cost may be very substantial.

6. All outcomes of interest in the analysis should be clearly identified, measured and valued.

The measure of outcome, effectiveness or benefit must always be appropriate to the intervention: for example, a measure of the effectiveness of an anti-depressant drug must be capable of registering changes in those aspects of health affected by depression. If the primary purpose of a therapy is to reduce the number of days with symptoms of gastro-oesophageal reflux disease, then effectiveness can be measured in terms of symptom-free days, and hence cost-effectiveness can be measured as the cost per symptom-free day. Similarly, if the purpose is to screen for cystic fibrosis, then cost-effectiveness could be measured in terms of the cost per case of cystic fibrosis detected.

But a very disease-specific measure of effectiveness is not particularly attractive from an economic perspective as it inevitably reduces the number of comparisons it is possible to make. A more general outcome measure often used in economic evaluations is the *life-year gained*. With this measure, the impact of any therapy *which affects mortality* can be measured in the same units. Hence the cost-effectiveness of a new neonatal intensive therapy unit in comparison with the existing service could be calculated as a cost per life-year gained. The cost-effectiveness of a new procedure for coronary bypass surgery in comparison with an existing procedure could also be calculated as a cost per life-year gained. The two results could then be compared to see whether it would be better to expand the budget for neonatal care or cardiology.

However, many interventions are not primarily intended to affect mortality, but rather mainly to affect quality of life. For example, a hip replacement operation is not chiefly concerned with improving someone's survival. To measure its effectiveness in terms of life-years gained would be seriously misleading. The concept used by economists to capture these quality-of-life effects is the QALY. If we can attach weights to particular health states, we can express most health outcomes in terms of QALYs, for they combine quality and quantity of life on the same scale. Figure 10.2 shows how two profiles of ill-health could be compared in terms of QALYs. The upper line shows a gain in quality of life and an extension in life expectancy (to the right of the dotted line), so that the shaded area represents the total gain in QALYs.

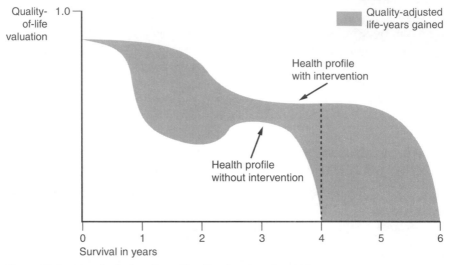

Figure 10.2   Hypothetical profiles of health-related quality of life.

We will examine different ways of calculating these values for a state of health or ill-health in Chapter 15. The key point is that the values are a numerical estimate of the value or *utility* which someone obtains from a health state, and therefore the study should state clearly whose values are being used (the public, patients, carers, 'experts'); the sample size; the method for eliciting values; the mean results and the variance.

7. Methods of obtaining estimates of effectiveness, resource use, unit costs, and quality-of-life valuations should be given alongside the sources of information.

As noted above, the process of estimating costs and effectiveness is done in steps: identification, measurement and, valuation. It is important to know how these steps were taken, so that the reader can assess the methods and quality of the data used. Questions to ask include: What sample sizes were used in measuring resource use? Were the unit costs used to value these resources obtained from reliable sources? Are they generalisable? Were the effectiveness data obtained from a controlled trial or overview of trials, or from some other source? How reliable are they? If quality-of-life valuations were used, how and where were they obtained?

C. RESULTS

8. The base case results in terms of costs, effectiveness, and incremental cost-effectiveness ratios, and the uncertainty surrounding them, should be clearly set out.

The end result of an economic evaluation is usually a cost-effectiveness ratio: that is, a cost per standard unit of outcome such as a life-year. However, when reporting results it is good practice to report the actual magnitude of cost and effect differences and not just the ratio. This makes it possible to see whether the actual cost and gain in health are very small or very large: if one intervention produced an additional 10 years of life expectancy per patient at a cost of £100 000, and another produced 5 weeks of additional life expectancy per patient at an additional cost of £1000, both would have a cost-effectiveness ratio of £10 000 per life-year gained, but would not necessarily be considered as equivalent by a decision-maker. One study of an adult tetanus immunisation programme (Balestra & Littenberg 1993) reported an incremental cost-effectiveness ratio of $143 138 per life-year saved, but in fact this ratio was obtained from an average cost of just 91 cents per patient and an average gain in life expectancy of only 2 minutes per patient! So it is good practice to give full information on costs and outcomes, and not just a cost-effectiveness ratio.

It is also crucial to note whether any reported differences in costs, effect or cost-effectiveness are statistically significant, or indeed whether the authors have reported the variance of these measures. It has become standard practice when reporting the results of clinical trials to give point estimates and their 95% confidence intervals. Similarly, information on costs should where possible report confidence intervals. Where cost estimates have not been obtained from a sample but have been modelled, or taken from the literature, or derived in some other way, the uncertainty surrounding any point estimate can still be conveyed by means of sensitivity analysis. The key assumptions can then be systematically varied to assess their impact on the results.

The same points hold with respect to the cost-effectiveness ratio, which should not be reported as a simple point estimate, but rather as a result which is subject to uncertainty concerning both the cost dimension and the effectiveness dimension.

9. The results should be placed in the context of other relevant economic evaluations.

Cost-effectiveness is a comparative methodology, the results of which make sense only in relation to other cost-effectiveness results. Therefore a range of other cost-effectiveness results should be quoted or referred to. This is especially important if the analyst wishes to draw a conclusion such as the intervention being studied 'is cost-effective compared to other uses of health care resources', or 'offers good value for money'. These other cost-effectiveness results should relate to areas that compete for resources with the intervention under investigation. This may be very broad, or may be confined to a specialty or age group or type of intervention. For example, if a proposed screening programme for colorectal cancer would have to be funded out of a screening budget, then it would be relevant to compare its cost-effectiveness with other screening programmes.

D. DISCUSSION

10. The relevance of the study for policy questions, and any ethical or distributive implications, should be discussed.

Policy makers have to balance a whole range of considerations, including legal, ethical and humanitarian concerns as well as evidence on cost-effectiveness. Suppose that an intervention was proven to be relatively cost-effective, but that it delivered most of its health gain to people who were already in very good health, or to a particular ethnic group. Or suppose it provided small health benefits to a large number of people, whereas other interventions against which it compared favourably provided large benefits to a small number of people. These implications of the intervention should be discussed.

In summary, any economic evaluation which satisfies the good practice guidelines set out above is likely to be a reliable source of information for evidence practice. In Chapter 15 we will consider in more detail how to interpret this evidence.

REFERENCES

Balestra D J, Littenberg B 1993 Should adult tetanus immunization be given as a single vaccination at age 65? Journal of General Internal Medicine 8:405–412
Canadian Coordinating Office for Health Technology Assessment 1997 Guidelines for economic evaluation of pharmaceuticals: Canada, 2nd edn. CCOHTA, Ottawa
Drummond M F, O'Brien B, Stoddart G L, Torrance G W 1997 Methods for the economic evaluation of health care programmes, 2nd edn. Oxford University Press, Oxford
Gerard K 1992 Cost utility in practice: a policy maker's guide to the state of the art. Health Policy 21:249–279
Gold M R, Siegel J E, Russell L B, Weinstein M C 1996 Cost-effectiveness in health and medicine. Oxford University Press, New York
Lieu T A, Cochi S L, Black S B, Halloran M E, Shinefield H R, Holmes S J, Wharton M, Washington A E 1994 Cost-effectiveness of a routine varicella vaccination program for US children. Journal of the American Medical Association 271(5):375–381
Udvarhelyi I S, Colditz A, Rai A, Epstein A M 1992 Cost-effectiveness and cost–benefit analyses in the medical literature. Are the methods being used correctly? Annals of Internal Medicine 116(3):238–244

11

Qualitative research

Kate Seers

Whilst reading through a recent journal, imagine you come across a piece of qualitative research that seems relevant to a clinical problem you have in your everyday practice. This article seems to throw light on something you have had in the back of your mind for some time. Perhaps the patient quotations are similar to comments you have been hearing, and you feel it could be a really useful paper.

For example, suppose you did a literature search to find out what types of medication were effective for alleviating chronic headache pain. You found several good studies that reported a specific treatment was effective. During your search, you also found a case study that looked interesting. You had not planned to use qualitative research in your review, but it caught your attention. The case study focused on one person's experience with this same pain medication that had been shown to be effective in previous studies. The article expressed a number of reservations about the treatment from the individual patient's point of view. It also gave the impression that there may be others who had similar reservations about their medication to the extent that they may not be taking it regularly. Does either study present the 'true' picture regarding the effectiveness of the medication? Could this example be typical of what other people were encountering with the treatment? Is it possible that people who were in the trials had not been taking the medication regularly because they had similar concerns?

You re-read the patient's account. You notice that there are a lot of other factors you need to know about the situation. Who talked to the patient? How long had the patient been in pain? What did the patient want from the treatment? What did the patient feel about side effects? You realise the case study suggests the need for a systematic qualitative study in this area.

But what is qualitative research, and how do you judge if it is any good?

This chapter will describe the various approaches to qualitative research and provide a framework for judging the quality and utility of qualitative research. If you are interested in undertaking qualitative research, suggestions for further reading are listed at the end of the chapter.

WHAT IS QUALITATIVE RESEARCH?

Qualitative research concentrates on people's experiences, attitudes and beliefs; their perceptions of a situation. It aims to generate an understanding of what is going on in an everyday setting. It can be used to generate new theory, describe a point of view, develop instruments, illustrate meanings, sensitise readers or try to understand phenomena (Forchuk & Roberts 1993). It may look at language (Silverman 1997). Qualitative research has been described as appropriate when we want to 'understand perceptions, motives and actions of individuals and organisations' (Boulton & Fitzpatrick 1997:83) and Fitzpatrick & Boulton (1994) stress that it involves conceptual development and analysis of underlying patterns. Popay & Williams (1998) argue very strongly that it is not the opposite of quantitative research and it is not just a set of techniques for collecting descriptive data: it has a theoretical foundation. This is important because this foundation is needed if knowledge generated from qualitative research is to be seen as legitimate. They see qualitative research as concerned with the 'negotiation and construction of meanings in social interaction' (Popay & Williams 1998:33–34).

Qualitative research can address such issues as: What is it like to have a certain condition, diagnosis, or type of care? What does it mean to the patient? For example, What is it like to have chronic pain? Qualitative research can be very good at providing the perspective of the patient and/or the health professional or other carer. The key is that the experience is explained and described by the participants, and they, not the researcher, provide the framework for what is important in that context.

Questions which can help the participant to explain their perspective might be:

- What has this experience been like?
- How has this experience made you feel?
- What do you think has helped you through this experience?
- Has anything made this experience more difficult?
- Why do you think that happened?
- Why did you do that?

Methods used in qualitative research include interviews (often semi- or unstructured), focus groups, observation (as a participant or as a non-participant) and examination of documentary evidence.

Qualitative research is a fairly new way of generating knowledge in health care. Many health-care professionals are more used to using quantitative research to inform their practice. The impetus for critically appraising quantitative research within evidence-based health care has come largely from clinical epidemiology and public health. Qualitative research has traditionally been outside that framework, and the whole process of assessing qualitative research is only just starting to be developed. However, Black (1994) argued for the value of qualitative research in health service research and Sackett & Wennberg (1997) stressed that the research question should determine the research design. The nursing profession has been publishing qualitative research for many years, and other disciplines such as medicine, occupational therapy, physiotherapy and health psychology are increasingly recognising its place in their research.

Some journals are specifically devoted to it, for example, Qualitative Health Research. The Cochrane Collaboration, which initially focused on quantitative research, especially RCTs, has widened its approach, and is considering setting up a Cochrane Methods Working Group to look at qualitative research (Cochrane Library 1998: Issue 3). The British Medical Journal frequently has articles on qualitative research and has published a book on this (Mays & Pope 1996). In 1998 much of an issue of the British Medical Journal was devoted to resistance to antibiotics. Alongside articles based on a range of quantitative approaches was a qualitative paper that aimed to increase our understanding of the culture of prescribing. It looked at general practitioners' and patients' perceptions of antibiotics for sore throats (Butler et al 1998) and found that prescribing decisions were greatly influenced by considerations of the doctor–patient relationship. This illustrates how a qualitative perspective can provide additional and different information from that obtained from more quantitative approaches, thus increasing our understanding of the total picture.

This suggests qualitative research is an appropriate form of research for health care and can provide useful information that contributes to the process of effective health care. Popay & Williams (1998) argue that barriers in the way of utilising the potential of qualitative research include the unequal social relationships of health research and the way the power and influence of different disciplines with their different views of knowledge may affect the collaboration of these disciplines. That is, the largely medical quantitative perspective is dominant and there may be a tendency to regard only knowledge generated from this approach as worthwhile knowledge. However, as qualitative research gains a higher profile in medical journals, and as a range of health professionals becomes familiar in its use and finds the knowledge it generates useful, these distinctions will very gradually become less marked. I hope that a greater understanding of a range of research methodologies, including their theoretical underpinnings and strengths and weaknesses, can only benefit patient care. This will start to happen as the wide range of clinical problems that practitioners and patients face is translated into research questions, answered using whichever research approach is most appropriate to that question.

Mutual understanding across these different approaches has not always been evident. The term 'qualitative research' just like 'quantitative research' covers a range of methodologies. Both approaches have in common the importance of asking a clear question, using a sensible methodology to answer that question, ensuring rigorous and systematic data collection and analysis and then explaining and interpreting the data and ensuring conclusions follow from the data. However, they are based on different ways of looking at the world and have different views of what constitutes valid knowledge and how it should be obtained. Thus they are based on different ways of knowing and produce different types of knowledge (*epistemological differences*). For example, quantitative research often produces numbers and looks at cause and effect to find out 'the truth'. Qualitative research is more likely to report on a variety of 'truths'.

Quantitative and qualitative research are also based on different ways of looking at reality or being (*ontological differences*). For example, quantitative research may look at very specific variables and one part of an experience, whereas qualitative research may look at the whole in context, and from the participants' perspectives. Quantitative research is often described as *deductive* (hypotheses are generated from theory) whereas qualitative research is described as *inductive* (theory is developed from the data). However, both can have elements of inductive and deductive approaches within them. For those readers who are interested in looking in more depth at the differences between qualitative and quantitative research and the different strengths and weaknesses of each approach, see Bryman (1988) and Seers (1994).

Whether qualitative research will be important to your clinical problem will depend on the question you are asking. For example, if you want to know whether relaxation is effective in reducing pain, an RCT is likely to be the appropriate design. However, if you want to know about patients' experiences of using relaxation (and this may address, for example, the barriers to using relaxation), then a qualitative approach is going to provide this sort of information. It could be that both questions are important to you, suggesting the use of both approaches.

There has been much debate about whether and how qualitative and quantitative approaches should be combined, and whether it is helpful to even use such distinctions. However, since they are commonly used, it may be helpful to look at how they can be used in a complementary way. Morgan (1998) points out that there are four basic combinations:

1. preliminary qualitative methods in a quantitative study
2. preliminary quantitative methods in a qualitative study
3. follow-up qualitative methods in a quantitative study.
4. follow-up quantitative methods in a qualitative study.

There are many different types of qualitative research, and an introductory text such as Burns & Grove (1997) can provide a useful overview. Very briefly, approaches you may come across in your reading include:

Phenomenology

This has its roots in a philosophical approach and looks at how people see their world. The term used is 'the lived experience'. Key early figures in this area include Husserl (1931) and Heidegger (1962). These texts are not easy going, and Koch (1995), Benner (1994) and Dreyfus (1991) offer more accessible accounts.

An example of a study in this area is Gravelle (1997) who looked at parents' experiences of caring for a child with progressive illness. She found that parents reported successive hardships and challenges, and they experienced cycles of defining and managing adversity, which were repeated with each important progressive change. This knowledge could be incorporated into the care of these children and their parents, to help them through these stages.

Another example is Ring & Danielson (1997) who studied patients' experiences of long-term oxygen therapy and reported four categories covering how patients coped. These included being restricted to time and place, being advantageous for the body, living one's own life rhythm and putting up with it in order to live. Having an understanding of these views of long-term oxygen therapy, which included social isolation, should enhance the ability of health-care professionals to deliver sensitive and tailored care to these patients.

Grounded theory

This comes from sociology (specifically symbolic interactionism). Here the aim is to generate theory from the data. Pioneers in this area are Glaser & Strauss (1967). Examples of studies in this area include Barclay et al (1997) who looked at women's experiences of early motherhood. They found becoming a mother was a difficult, multi-factorial process and highlighted six different categories: being overwhelmed, being unready, feeling drained, feeling alone, experiencing a feeling of loss and gaining confidence. These findings suggest how health-care professionals supporting these women could help them through this challenging time of change.

Wilson (1997), who studied the transition to nursing home life for older adults, identified three phases: feeling overwhelmed, adjusting and initial acceptance. Again, an understanding of this process gives prompts to the assessment and planning of care to make this process as smooth as possible for older people entering nursing homes.

Ethnography

This has been developed from anthropology and looks at behaviour within a culture (which can include a society or a social group). An early worker in this field was Mead (1935). Examples of ethnographic research include Barroso (1997) on becoming a long-term survivor of AIDs and Savage (1995) who explored the notion of 'closeness' in nurse–patient relationships. Barroso (1997) found five overlapping dimensions of adapting that were normalising, focusing on living, taking care of one's self, being in relation to others and triumphing. Bouthillette (1998) argues that this suggests a possible intervention for nurses of focusing on the positive rather than the negative. It may be that being aware of these five dimensions could help you plan your discussions with similar patients. The closeness identified by Savage (1995) in nurse–patient relationships was found to be affected by adequate resources being available to support the nurses. This study has implications for the planning of care and questions the basing of nursing care on 'closeness' if the resources are not available to sustain such patient-focused care.

These approaches all try to build up a picture of what is happening; they interpret.

Hermeneutics

This is a perspective that aims to create a dialogue where participants' and observers' meanings and interpretations interact, producing what Gadamer (1993) refers to as a 'fusion of horizons', or a new understanding. It aims to offer an account of both the world as understood by those participating in it, and the barriers that might prevent such an understanding being achieved. Understanding is in constant movement, from the whole to the parts and from the parts to the whole. This has been termed the 'hermeneutical circle of understanding' (Heidegger 1990). For example, Smith (1998) used a hermeneutic phenomenological approach to look at the experience of people with drinking problems, and found they described their experience of suffering as a spiralling, vicious vortex.

Critical theory

This has a different approach, as it aims specifically to increase people's understanding of their situation and through this they initiate change. Emancipation or empowerment are two words often seen in this type of research.

One influential figure in this approach is Habermas (1985) (see also Fay (1987) and Dunne (1993) for more details). Much feminist research would come into this category; see, for example, Webb (1993) for more information.

Some of the traditionally more interpretative types of the research listed above may also adopt a critical theory approach. Some action research can be described as adopting this perspective, for example, Titchen & Binnie (1993). They looked at a change from traditional, standardised nursing to patient-centred nursing via primary nursing. Their action research strategy for this change included 'working towards the democratisation of health care through the emancipation of nurses who are, traditionally, trapped in a bureaucratic nursing hierarchy and in oppressive doctor–nurse relationships' (Titchen & Binnie 1993:25). Their other strategies included introducing innovation and facilitating change; helping practitioners to research their own practice; facilitating professional learning and reflective practice, and generating and testing theory.

Some qualitative research does not use a methodological framework which fits into one of these types of design. For example, Armstrong et al (1996) conducted semi-structured interviews with general practitioners to look at their reasons for changing prescribing patterns. They reported the findings without a theoretical foundation. As discussed earlier, Popay & Williams (1998) argue a theoretical foundation is needed if knowledge generated from qualitative research is to be seen as legitimate.

Qualitative findings, partly because they use quotations that are sometimes very powerful, are often very accessible to the reader, and it is important to ensure the same level of critical appraisal is undertaken as with any other type of research design.

COMMON CRITICISMS OF QUALITATIVE RESEARCH

Before the next section addressing 'what is a good qualitative study?', some common criticisms of qualitative research will be considered. These criticisms often stem from applying quantitative criteria to qualitative research, such as 'This research is subjective, not reliable and cannot be generalised.' This is the sort of comment you may hear when qualitative research is being discussed by those unused to this approach.

Bias

When you are appraising quantitative research, you are looking for design features that minimise bias. In a qualitative study, 'bias' is treated rather differently. The whole point of the study is usually to look specifically at the experience of the participant and this process will be influenced by the researcher's perspective. What is key here is that this perspective is clearly recorded. Since many of the decisions will be subjective, a clear, documented rationale for all decisions made is crucial. This is sometimes referred to as a *decision trail*. This is linked to auditability (sometimes known as trustworthiness), the qualitative term similar to reliability.

Auditability (trustworthiness)/reliability

Here you are not looking for someone else to get exactly the same results in a similar setting, because it is acknowledged that the researcher's perceptions and background influence the questions asked, the data obtained and how it is interpreted. (This influence is also quite possible in quantitative research, but is not usually acknowledged.) What is important is that someone else can follow your decision trail.

Fittingness/generalisability

Generalisability is sometimes referred to as *external validity* in quantitative research and as *fittingness* in qualitative research.

A representative sample from which one can generalise to other populations is important in quantitative research. In qualitative research, participants are not usually selected as part of a random sample, but because they have the specific characteristic(s) the researcher is interested in addressing.

Fitzpatrick & Boulton (1994) stress the need to ensure the sample contains a full range of possible observations so concepts and categories provide a reasonable conceptualisation of the subject. They describe the conceptual generalisation that takes place in qualitative research. So you are looking for generalising from the findings to a theoretical body of knowledge (or creating new knowledge) rather than to a population.

Qualitative research should give a description to allow you to decide whether the findings might be relevant to people for whom you care. One of the benefits of this type of research is that you may become aware of issues you had not considered or had not had time to concentrate on, and then your increased sensitivity to these issues means you can test them out in practice. For example, if you care for people who are long-term survivors of AIDS, and you read Barroso (1997) it may be that knowing they had five dimensions of adapting (normalising, focusing on living, taking care of oneself, being in relation to others and triumphing) could help you plan your discussions with your patients.

Credibility/validity

Are you measuring/understanding what you think you are measuring/understanding? This is known as *internal validity* in quantitative research and as *credibility* in qualitative research. Both approaches may want to maximise validity by triangulation. That is, obtaining data from a range of sources. In qualitative research, respondent validation, where the researcher checks with the participants whether they agree with the researcher's analysis, can be used, although as Fitzpatrick & Boulton (1994) point out, participants may have reasons for not agreeing with the interpretation of events, which in themselves can be revealing.

WHAT IS A GOOD QUALITATIVE STUDY?

Popay et al (1998) outline why it is important to have criteria to evaluate qualitative research.

- It may be judged as inferior by those who see RCTs as the gold standard.
- There is a need to understand lay and professional decision-making.
- Questions are proposed that cannot be explored or explained by RCTs.

- It is necessary if you want to carry out a systematic review of qualitative research.
- Researchers using qualitative research in the health service may have little or no familiarity with disciplines in which the methods were developed and the assumptions underlying them. They feel this limits the capacity to maximise the potential within these approaches.
- Calls from qualitative research (Altheide & Johnson 1994) underline the need to look at the wider methodological and epistemological context within which the methods are applied, as well as the actual methods used.

Questions to help with critical appraisal

Various different sets of questions are available for helping you to undertake a critical appraisal of qualitative research (Beck 1993, Boulton & Fitzpatrick 1997, CASP 1998, Forchuk & Roberts 1993, Greenhalgh & Taylor 1997, Kuckelmann-Cobb & Nelson-Hagemaster 1987, Locke et al 1998, Mays & Pope 1996, Medical Sociology Group 1996, Miles & Huberman 1994, Popay et al 1998).

Framework guide to critical appraisal

Popay et al (1998) will be used here as a framework to guide critical appraisal. They argue that there is no absolute list of criteria, but recognise the need for some sort of framework, whilst acknowledging that this framework will require further development.

This framework consists of a list of numbered areas for consideration, followed by a question or questions to tap that area.

1. Privileging subjective meaning

Q. Does this research, as reported, illuminate the subjective meaning, actions and context of those being researched?

This is seen as a fundamental question (which they term a *primary marker*).

The research should show how behaviours are viewed from within a culture, group or society.

Thus the subjective meaning of the participants should be retained during analysis and reporting of the findings. The explanations and views of the participants should be presented from their own point of view and nested within their own context. The researcher should use direct quotations, accounts and stories where possible to illustrate that insights have been gained from the data analysis.

They argue that an explanation that is meaningful may help us understand why something has happened or is the way it is (Popay et al 1998: 345).

The research must give lay knowledge equal worth to other knowledge. So here you want to establish whether the research gives lay knowledge equal worth to the knowledge of the researcher and the potential users of the research.

The researcher may value personal analysis and views over those of the participants. Dissenting views may be minimised or ignored to support the position of those in control of resources and decision-making. The process of politicising the findings devalues both the researcher and the participants and renders the results less useful in terms of their ability to inform policy. Popay et al (1998) argue that lay knowledge has the potential to address key policy issues that have eluded the efforts of policy-makers. Understanding why people act as they do (e.g. non-compliance with prescribed drug or other treatment regimens) is important if any improvement is to be made. Thus emphasis is given to the views and explanations of the participants, and Popay et al describe this as a position that privileges the lay view.

2. Evidence of responsiveness to social context and flexibility of design

Q. Is there any evidence of the adaptation and responsiveness of the research design to the circumstances and real-life social settings met during the course of the study?

Here they highlight that qualitative research does not have a standardised protocol to be followed, but a hallmark of good qualitative methodology is its variability rather than its standardisation. Adaptation and redesign should be evident in the report. Another point to bear in mind is that sampling, data collection, analysis and interpretation should not be separate in qualitative research, but part of an iterative process. The experience of data collection and analysis, for example, may lead the researcher to revisit the original participants to obtain more points of view, or to include more people in the sample. At a further point in the research, findings from preliminary data analysis may lead the researcher to revisit the data and look at it from a different perspective.

3. Evidence of theoretical or purposive sampling

Q. Does the sample produce the type of knowledge necessary to understand the structures and processes within which the individuals or situations are located?

Here randomness and representativeness are of less concern than relevance. The sampling strategy needs to be appropriate for the research question and the environment in which the data are being collected. Often insights gained from the first 'round' of data collection suggest to the researcher whether to continue sampling to confirm or refute preliminary findings.

In a paper you need to look for an adequate description of a theoretically or purposefully selected sample. There is much debate about the definition of these two types of sampling, and whether they are different (see Coyne 1997). One definition of theoretical sampling is 'the process of data collection whereby the researcher simultaneously collects, codes and analyses the data in order to decide what data to collect next' (Coyne 1997: 625). Theoretical sampling methods work well in environments where researchers have the freedom to return many times to the research setting. They are also essential for research studies where new theories are being developed.

This contrasts with purposive sampling which is usually based on an a priori decision about the selection of informants by the researcher to obtain as many perspectives as possible. Purposive sampling is often used when researchers have limited access to the research environment, or limited time in which to conduct the study. It is also used when there is already an existing body of knowledge, or a theory that has been generated, from a particular population. Thus prior knowledge about the range and diversity of perspectives can be used to make an informed decision about the types of people or views that need to be included in the sample. So you are looking to see whether a range of appropriate individuals has been selected to fit the aims of the study.

When using either purposive or theoretical sampling, the researcher must ensure that all the data relevant to the research question are collected (*data saturation*). In theoretical sampling, this will mean the population is revisited until emerging theories are either confirmed or refuted. In purposive sampling, this will mean that a wide range of members of the population is consulted until no new views are obtained.

4. Evidence of adequate description

Q. Is the description provided detailed enough to allow the researcher or reader to interpret the meaning and context of what is being researched?

They point out that it is not just depth but purpose that is important. So you are looking for not just what happened, but the whole process and context. This could include ethical issues, such as whether consent of participants, confidentiality and risks/benefits have been addressed.

The description of the research needs to include the original reasons for conducting the research, the political, policy and social context in which the investigation is being conducted, the bias of the researcher, the population setting, and if possible the attitudes of the participants toward the research. This type of 'rich description' enables the reader to gain a better understanding and interpretation of the research.

5. Evidence of data quality

Q. How are the different sources of knowledge about the same issue compared and contrasted?

They argue that this is more than just triangulation where you are looking for confirmation of accounts, but extends into different facets of the experience being investigated. This could include discussion of the number of participants and data saturation, where additional participants are giving similar rather than new information, and this links back to point 3 on this appraisal checklist.

Another related question in this section is:

Q. Are subjective perceptions and experiences treated as knowledge in their own right?

When analysing and reporting the research, the researcher must distinguish between the knowledge of the participants, the knowledge the researcher originally brought to the project, and the insights the researcher has gained along the way. If this distinction is made in the reporting of the results, then readers will be able to separate accounts of participants' views from the views of the researcher, and regard them as knowledge in their own right. Thus it should be clear what is description of the data obtained (such as the participants' accounts, and the setting) and what are the researcher's views and analysis.

Addressing the influence of the researcher, Popay & Williams (1998) argue that the question is not 'are the data biased?' as the researcher will be shaping the data. The question is how far has the researcher made clear the process by which the researcher has collected, analysed and presented the data. They point out that all data is the result of interaction, and as such the researcher must be extensively involved if the intricacies of the accounts and situations are to be adequately described.

Other issues to consider here include some of those suggested by Forchuk & Roberts (1993), which look at whether the descriptions of informants/participants, context and researcher were adequate. For example, was the researcher's perspective declared early? The researcher's level of participation and preconceptions/perspectives about the phenomenon need to be made explicit. The reader can then take this perspective into account when looking at the study results.

Were data analysed systematically? For example, were themes identified, and if so was this done manually or using a computer programme (such as Nudist®).

How many researchers analysed the data? Although you would not necessarily expect two researchers to come up with exactly the same categories for every piece of data, in, for example, a transcript, it is useful to have more than one person undertake this, to ensure themes are not missed.

6. Evidence of theoretical and conceptual adequacy

Q. How does the research move from a description of the data, through quotations of examples, to an analysis and interpretation of the meaning and significance of it?

This is looking at interpretative validity, where the analytical path is explicitly described. It should be clear how the phenomenon, situation or event that is being researched related to the theory or insights that are being generated by the researcher. In other words, is it clear how the researcher arrived at the conclusions, and do the conclusions seem justified by the data?

7. Potential for assessing typicality

Q. What claims are being made for the generalisability of the findings to either other bodies of knowledge or to other populations or groups?

Are the findings generalisable? They say 'the aim is to make logical generalisations to a theoretical understanding of a similar class of phenomena rather than a probabilistic generalisation to a population' (Popay et al 1998: 348). For example, Wilson's (1997) grounded theory study found that older adults went through three phases of adjusting to a permanent nursing home admission (feeling overwhelmed, adjustment and initial acceptance). This does not predict how older people will react in this situation, but suggests reactions that might typically occur in this situation.

Popay & Williams (1998) argue that confidence in typicality can be enhanced by use of official and non-official statistics, policy documents and other pieces of research.

8. Relevance to policy

Q. Is the relevance of research to a variety of different stakeholders clearly indicated?

The research needs to have implications for both practice and policy.

It is interesting that despite Popay et al's (1998) argument that qualitative research should be linked to a theoretical basis, this does not form one of the questions. This is included in Mays & Pope's checklist (1996:18).

I hope this has given you a flavour and a few signposts for starting to critically appraise qualitative research articles. It might be helpful to look at the other critical appraisal checklists which have been developed in this area (see p. **119**): it is an ongoing development and all are subject to revision and fine tuning. I hope that as you critically evaluate qualitative research, you will start to separate the wheat from the chaff and start to feel comfortable that high quality qualitative research can inform your practice. You may find that one of your particular clinical problems is such that it needs to be answered by qualitative research. Linking with a qualitative researcher and using these criteria as you design your own qualitative research may help you produce qualitative research that others will want to use.

Acknowledgement

Many thanks to Janet Harris for her helpful comments and to other colleagues who commented on drafts of this chapter.

REFERENCES

Altheide D, Johnson J 1994 Criteria for assessing interpretative validity in qualitative research. In: Denzin N, Lincoln Y (eds) Handbook of qualitative research. Sage, Thousand Oaks, ch 30, p 485–499
Armstrong D, Reyburn H, Jones R 1996 A study of general practitioners' reasons for changing their prescribing behaviour. British Medical Journal 312:949–952
Barclay L, Everitt L, Rogan F et al 1997 Becoming a mother – an analysis of women's experience of early motherhood. Journal of Advanced Nursing 25:719–728
Barroso J 1997 Reconstructing my life: becoming a long term survivor of AIDS. Qualitative Health Research 7:57–74
Beck C T 1993 Qualitative research: the evaluation of its credibility, fittingness, and auditability. Western Journal of Nursing Research 15(2):263–266
Benner P 1994 Interpretative phenomenology. Sage, Thousand Oaks
Black N 1994 Why we need qualitative research. Journal of Epidemiology and Community Health 48:425–426
Boulton M, Fitzpatrick R 1997 Evaluating qualitative research. Evidence Based Health Policy and Management 1(4):83–85
Bouthillette F 1998 Commentary on Barroso. Evidence Based Nursing 1(1):32
Bryman A 1988 Quantity and quality in social research. Unwin Hyman, London
Burns N, Grove S K 1997 The practice of nursing research. Conduct, critique and utilisation, 3rd edn. W B Saunders, Philadelphia
Butler C G, Rollnick S, Pill R, Maggs-Rapport F, Stott N 1998 Understanding the culture of prescribing: a qualitative study of general practitioners' and patients' perceptions of antibiotics for sore throats. British Medical Journal 317:637–642
CASP (Critical Appraisal Skills Programme) 1998 10 questions to help you make sense of qualitative research. CASP, Oxford (Contact: CASP Office, Institute of Health Sciences, Old Road, Headington, Oxford OX3 7LF; http://www.ihs.ox.ac.uk/casp/qualitative.html)
Cochrane Library 1998 Issue 3. Update Software, London
Coyne I T 1997 Sampling in qualitative research. Purposeful and theoretical sampling; merging or clear boundaries? Journal of Advanced Nursing 26:623–630
Dreyfus H L 1991 Being-in-the-world. A commentary on Heidegger's Being and time, Division I. MIT Press, Cambridge, Massachusetts
Dunne J 1993 Back to the rough ground: 'Phronesis' and 'techne' in modern philosophy and in Aristotle. University of Notre Dame Press, Notre Dame
Fay B 1987 Critical social science. Liberation and its limits. Polity Press, Cambridge
Fitzpatrick R, Boulton M 1994 Qualitative methods for assessing health care. Quality in Health Care 3(2):107–113
Forchuk C, Roberts J 1993 How to critique qualitative research articles. Canadian Journal of Nursing Research 25(4):47–56
Gadamer H G 1993 Truth and Method. Sheed & Ward, London
Glaser B G, Strauss A L 1967 The discovery of grounded theory: strategies for qualitative research. Aldine, Chicago
Gravelle A M 1997 Caring for a child with progressive illness during the complex chronic phase: parents' experiences of facing adversity. Journal of Advanced Nursing 25:738–745

Greenhalgh T, Taylor R 1997 How to read a paper. Papers that go beyond numbers (qualitative research). British Medical Journal 315:740–743

Habermas J 1985 Die neue Unübersichtlichkeit. Suhrkramp, Frankfurt (translation in The Habermas Reader 1996 Polity Press, Cambridge)

Heidegger M 1962 Being and time. Harper & Row, New York (original publication in German 1927)

Heidegger M 1990 Being and time. Blackwell, Oxford

Husserl E 1931 Ideas. General introduction to pure phenomenology. Allen Lane, London

Koch T 1995 Interpretative approaches in nursing research: the influence of Husserl and Heidegger. Journal of Advanced Nursing 21:827–836

Kuckelmann – Cobb A, Nelson-Hagemaster J 1987 Ten criteria for evaluating qualitative research proposals. Journal of Nursing Education 26 (4):138–143

Locke L F, Silverman S J, Spirduso W W 1998 Reading and understanding research. Sage, Thousand Oaks

Mays N, Pope C 1996 Qualitative research in health care. British Medical Journal, London

Mead M 1935 Sex and temperament in three primitive societies. Morrow, New York

Medical Sociology Group 1996 Criteria for the evaluation of qualitative research papers. Medical Sociology News 22 (1):68–71

Miles M B, Huberman A M 1994 Qualitative data analysis, 2nd edn. Sage, Thousand Oaks, ch 10, p 277–280

Morgan D L 1998 Practical strategies for combining qualitative and quantitative methods: applications to health research. Qualitative Health Research 8(3):362–376

Popay J, Rogers A, Williams G 1998 Rationale and standards for the systematic review of qualitative literature in health services research. Qualitative Health Research 8 (3):341–351

Popay J, Williams G 1998 Qualitative research and evidence based health care. Journal of The Royal Society of Medicine 91 (Suppl 35):32–37

Ring L, Danielson E 1997 Patients' experiences of long term oxygen therapy. Journal of Advanced Nursing 26:337–344

Sackett D L, Wennberg J E 1997 Choosing the best research design for each question. Editorial. British Medical Journal 315:1636

Savage J 1995 Nursing intimacy: An ethnographic approach to nurse–patient interaction. Scutari Press, Harrow

Seers K 1994 Qualitative and quantitative research. Surgical Nurse 7(6): 4–6

Silverman D (ed) 1997 Qualitative research. Theory, method and practice. Sage, London

Smith B A 1998 The problem drinker's lived experience of suffering: an exploration using hermeneutic phenomenology. Journal of Advanced Nursing 27:213–222

Titchen A, Binnie A 1993 A unified action research strategy. Nursing Educational Action Research 1(1):25–33

Webb C 1993 Feminist research: definitions, methodology, methods and evaluation. Journal of Advanced Nursing 18:416–423

Wilson S A 1997 The transition to nursing home life: a comparison of planned and unplanned admissions. Journal of Advanced Nursing 26:864–871

Additional reading for those interested in finding out more about qualitative research

Burns N, Grove S K 1997 The practice of nursing research. Conduct, critique and utilisation, 3rd edn. W B Saunders, Philadelphia

Denzin N K, Lincoln Y S (eds) 1994 Handbook of qualitative research. Sage, Thousand Oaks

Flick U 1998 An introduction to qualitative research. Sage, London

Holloway I 1997 Basic concepts for qualitative research. Blackwell Science, Oxford

Miles M B, Huberman A M 1994 Qualitative data analysis, 2nd edn. Sage, Thousand Oaks, ch 10, p 277–280

Silverman D (ed) 1997 Qualitative research. Theory, method and practice. Sage, London

12

Critical appraisal of clinical guidelines

Robin Snowball

Another piece of paper lands on your desk: yet another guideline about a condition clinicians have been treating for years. It is tempting to throw it away but it may contain important information! How can you tell whether it is worth reading in the first place? It may be a summary of the evidence put together succinctly and clearly and may (if implemented) positively affect patient care. On the other hand, it may represent out-of-date opinions and, if implemented, potentially harm patients. We need a guide which can be used quickly to assess the quality of guidelines.

Clinical guidelines should be 'systematically developed statements to assist practitioner and patients' decisions about appropriate health care for specific clinical circumstances' (Field & Lohr 1990). They are a form of literature intended to be immediately usable for clinical decision-making and to improve care. Grimshaw & Russell (1993), for example, systematically reviewed 59 evaluations of clinical guidelines and their effect on practice, and found significant improvements in the process and outcomes of care following their introduction. However, it is always necessary to question the process of development of a guideline, and to determine to what extent it is actually based on sound and up-to-date research evidence of an appropriate kind and range.

This is a burgeoning field, as you would expect. In the Select List of Information Resources at the end of Chapter 3, addresses of Web sites for finding guidelines are given. (A Web search using the search engine OMNI, also in the Select List, with subject search terms or 'guidelines' and 'guideline' will also find related sites, organisations and publications of interest.)

In this chapter we will present a model critical appraisal instrument – 'Appraisal Instrument for Clinical Guidelines' (Cluzeau et al 1997). The instrument was developed and tested (on some 80 guidelines) by the Health Care Evaluation Unit at St George's Hospital Medical School in London in collaboration with the Health Services Research Unit at Aberdeen University, the Department of General Practice at St Bartholomew's Hospital, London, and the Royal London School of Medicine and Dentistry, Queen Mary and Westfield College.

The instrument provides a 'transparent and standardised method 'for critical appraisal of existing clinical guidelines, as well as a checklist for the development of new ones. It will be updated regularly to keep pace with the quality of clinical guidelines being developed. The current version (Version 1) is expected to be revised in 1999. Further details about the instrument and the research programme are available on the St George's Health Care Evaluation Web site: http://www.sghms.ac.uk/phs/hceu/.

Permission to quote from and to reproduce the instrument has been very kindly given by Françoise Cluzeau (e-mail: F. Cluzeau@SGHMS.ac.uk) of the Health Care Evaluation Unit at St Georges, who welcomes comments relating to it. It is produced as a very attractive and easy-to-use, A4-size questionnaire booklet, in a folder which also contains a User Guide which gives descriptions of terms used in the questions, notes which ensure that questions are consistently interpreted, and much useful information relating to assessment of guidelines. You can view it on the web site.

The instrument contains 37 questions – divided into three 'dimensions', sub-divided by headings – which require 'Yes/No' (or 'Not applicable') responses:

DIMENSION 1 Rigour of development (Questions 1–20)

Responsibility for guidelines development

Is the agency responsible for the development of the guidelines clearly identified?
Was external funding or other support received for developing the guidelines?
If external funding or support was received, is there evidence that the potential biases of the funding body(ies) were taken into account?

Guidelines development group

Is there a description of the individuals who were involved in the guidelines development group?
If so, did the group contain representatives of all key disciplines?

Identification and interpretation of evidence

Is there a description of the sources of information used to select the evidence upon which the recommendations are based?
If so, are the sources of information adequate?
Is there a description of the method(s) used to interpret and assess the strength of the evidence?
If so, is (are) the method(s) for rating the evidence satisfactory?

Formulation of recommendations

Is there a description of the methods used to formulate the recommendations?
If so, are the methods satisfactory?

Is there an indication of how the views of interested parties not on the panel were taken into account?
Is there an explicit link between the major recommendations and the level of supporting evidence?

Peer review

Were the guidelines independently reviewed prior to their publication/ release?
If so, is explicit information given about methods and how comments were addressed?
Were the guidelines piloted?
If the guidelines were piloted, is explicit information given about the methods used and the results adopted?

Updating

Is there a mention of a date for reviewing or updating the guidelines?
Is the body responsible for the reviewing and updating clearly identified?

Overall assessment of the development process

Overall, have the potential biases of guidelines development been adequately dealt with?

DIMENSION 2 Context and content (Questions 21–32)

Objectives

Are the reasons for developing the guidelines clearly stated?
Are the objectives of the guidelines clearly defined?

Context

Is there a satisfactory description of the patients to which the guidelines are meant to apply?
Is there a description of the circumstances (clinical or non-clinical) in which exceptions might be made in using the guidelines?
Is there an explicit statement of how patients' preferences should be taken into account in applying the guidelines?

Clarity

Do the guidelines describe the condition to be detected, treated or prevented in unambiguous terms?

Are the different possible options for management of the condition clearly stated in the guidelines?
Are the recommendations clearly presented?

Likely costs and benefits

Is there an adequate description of the health benefits that are likely to be gained from the recommended management?
Is there an adequate description of the potential harms or risks that may occur as a result of the recommended management?
Is there an estimate of the costs or expenditures likely to incur from the recommended management?
Are the recommendations supported by the estimated benefits, harms and costs of the intervention?

DIMENSION 3 Application (Questions 33–37)

Guidelines dissemination and implementation

Does the guidelines document suggest possible methods for dissemination and implementation?

Monitoring of guidelines/clinical audit

Does the guidelines document specify criteria for monitoring compliance?
Does the guidelines document identify clear standards or targets?
Does the guidelines document define measurable outcomes that can be monitored?

National guidelines only

Does the guidelines document identify key elements which need to be considered by local guidelines groups?

REFERENCES

Cluzeau F, Littlejohns P, Grimshaw J, Feder G 1997 Appraisal instrument for clinical guidelines: version 1. St George's Hospital Medical School, London. (Available from Mrs Loretta Hall, Health Care Evaluation Unit, Dept of Public Health Sciences, St George's Hospital Medical School, London SW17 0RE; Tel. 0181 725 5428; Fax 0181 725 3584; e-mail L.Hall@SGHMS.ac.uk) URL: http://www.sghms.ac.uk/phs/hceu/index.htm

Field M J, Lohr K N (eds) 1990 Clinical practice guidelines: directions for a new program. Committee to Advise the Public Health Service on Clinical Practice Guidelines, Institute of Medicine. National Academy Press, Washington DC
Grimshaw J M, Russell I T 1993 Effect of clinical guidelines on medical practice: a systematic review of rigorous evaluations. Lancet 342 (8883):1317–1322

13

Is this test effective?

Jonathan Mant

Tests are performed in health care for a variety of different reasons. They may be used to establish whether or not someone has a disease, to monitor response to therapy in someone with a disease, to inform treatment decisions in someone with known disease, to assess prognosis or to assess someone's risk of developing a disease. The criteria with which you would assess if a test is effective will depend upon the purpose for which the test is being performed. In this chapter, we shall focus on using tests to help us decide whether or not someone has a disease.

DECIDING WHETHER OR NOT SOMEONE HAS A DISEASE

In an ideal world, a positive test would mean that someone has a disease, and a negative test would mean that the person does not have a disease. Unfortunately, this is not always the case. As we saw in Chapter 6, how we appraise a diagnostic test is to compare its performance with a gold standard, which aims to represent 'the truth'. When a test is carried out, there are four possible outcomes[1]:

1. The test can correctly detect disease that is present (a *true positive* result).
2. The test can detect disease when it is really absent (a *false positive* result).
3. The test can correctly identify that someone does not have a disease (a *true negative* result).
4. The test can identify someone as being free of a disease when it is really present (a *false negative* result).

These possible outcomes are illustrated in Table 13.1. Given that a test may potentially mislead us if we get a false positive or a false negative result, we need to have some way of characterising how accurate the test really is.

1. HOW ACCURATE IS THE TEST?

The traditional way in which the accuracy of a test is characterised is in terms of *sensitivity* and *specificity*. The sensitivity reflects how good the test is at picking up people with disease, while the specificity reflects how good

---

[1]To keep things simple, for the time being we are ignoring 'borderline' test results, but we will come back to these later in the chapter.

Table 13.1   Possible outcomes of a diagnostic test

		'Truth' Disease present	Disease absent	Totals
Test result	Positive	a true positive	b false positive	a + b
	Negative	c false negative	d true negative	c + d
	Totals	a + c	b + d	a + b + c + d

Sensitivity = a/(a + c)
Specificity = d/(b + d)

Positive predictive value = a/(a + b)
Negative predictive value = d/(c + d)

Prevalence = (a + c)/(a + b + c + d)

the test is at identifying people without the disease. What these terms mean can best be understood by way of an example.

Let us consider mammography as a screening test for breast cancer. In the UK, women aged 50 to 64 are invited at 3-yearly intervals for a special X-ray of the breast, called a mammogram, to ascertain whether they might have breast cancer. In one study, the sensitivity of mammography was reported as 88% and the specificity as 93% (Garvican & Littlejohns 1996). What does this mean? Well, the sensitivity of 88% means that for every 100 women with breast cancer who have a mammogram, 88 of them will have a positive (i.e. abnormal) test result. The specificity of 93% means that for every 100 women without breast cancer who have a mammogram, 93 of them will have a negative (i.e. normal) test. The derivation of sensitivity and specificity is shown algebraically in Table 13.1, and using breast cancer screening data in Table 13.2. Sensitivity may then be defined as the proportion of people with disease that have a positive test result, and specificity may be defined as the proportion of people without disease that have a negative test result.

What does the test result mean for an individual patient?

The problem with using sensitivity and specificity as a way of summarising test accuracy is that they are difficult to interpret for individual patients. What the patient wants to know, as does the health-care professional looking after that patient, might be put something like this: 'Does this positive test mean I have breast cancer?' Or, for someone who has a normal test result: 'Does this negative test mean I do not have breast cancer?' The answers to these questions may be found by looking at Table 13.2. This shows that there were 1000 women who had a positive test. Of these, 90 actually had breast cancer, and 910 did not have breast cancer. Therefore, the chance that someone with a positive test actually has breast cancer is 90/1000, or 9%. In other words, the answer to the first question is: 'No, you

Table 13.2 Accuracy of breast cancer screening by mammography in healthy women

		'Truth' Breast cancer present	Breast cancer absent	Totals
Mammography result	Positive	90	910	1000
	Negative	12	12 090	12 102
	Totals	102	13 000	13 102

Sensitivity = 90/102 = 88%
Specificity = 12 090/13 000 = 93%

Positive predictive value = 90/1000 = 9%
Negative predictive value = 12 090/12 102 = 99.9%

Prevalence = 102/13 102 = 0.78%

Adapted from Garvican & Littlejohns 1996.

probably do not have breast cancer. For every hundred women like yourself with a positive mammogram, only nine will actually turn out to have breast cancer.' This figure of 9% is referred to as the *positive predictive value*, and its algebraic derivation is shown in Table 13.1.

With regard to the second question, Table 13.2 shows that of 12 102 people who had a negative mammogram, 12 090 really did not have breast cancer, and only 12 did. Therefore, the chance that someone with a negative test does not have breast cancer is 12 090/12 102, or 99.9%. This is referred to as the *negative predictive value*. Therefore, the answer to the second question is: 'Yes, this negative test means that it is very unlikely that you have breast cancer. For every 1000 women like yourself with a negative mammogram, only one has breast cancer.'

Therefore, from the perspective of the individual, breast cancer screening seems very good at ruling out disease if the test is normal, but not very good at diagnosing disease in that 91% of people with a positive test will turn out not to have breast cancer. You get no hint of this from the sensitivity and the specificity, which both sound quite impressive. Why then, do we not use negative and positive predictive values as our standard way of reporting test accuracy, since it is these values that the patient and the health-care professional really need to know?

Effect of prevalence on predictive value

The problem is that predictive value is dependent upon how common the disease is in the population that is being tested. In a population of healthy women aged 50 to 64, breast cancer is in fact fairly uncommon. You can see from Table 13.2 that in the study we referred to earlier only 102 (90 true positives and 12 false negatives) out of 13 102 women tested actually turned out to have breast cancer. This represents 0.78% of the population tested. This can be referred to as the *prevalence* of the disease in the population. Prevalence is defined as the proportion of people with disease in a defined population at a given point in time. The algebraic derivation of prevalence in relation to a diagnostic test is shown in Table 13.1.

Suppose we had performed mammography on a different population where we would expect a higher prevalence of breast cancer, for example women referred to a surgical out-patient clinic with a breast lump. Of course, mammography would not usually be used in this circumstance nowadays, but has been used in the past in this way. Table 13.3 shows the results of a study reported in 1983 looking at mammography in women with breast lumps (Winchester et al 1983). The prevalence of breast cancer in this population is 36%. You can see that the specificity (95%) and sensitivity (76%) of the test in this population of women are not very different from when it was performed in healthy women (Table 13.2). However, the positive predictive value has changed dramatically, and is now 89%. This is much higher than the 9% using the same test in a population with a low prevalence (Table 13.2). This demonstrates that the positive predictive value of a test is dependent upon the prevalence of disease in the population being tested. Conversely, the sensitivity and specificity of the test do **not** change when performed in a low prevalence (healthy women) or a high prevalence population (women with breast lumps).

This is not to say that sensitivity and specificity are always constant. It is just that they are not affected by prevalence. We will look at what sort of things might make sensitivity and specificity change later in the chapter.

This effect of prevalence on positive predictive value is further illustrated in Table 13.4, which shows how well the same test, the CAGE questionnaire for identifying alcoholism, performs in a primary care population and in a hospital population.

Table 13.3   Accuracy of mammography in diagnosing breast cancer in women with breast lumps

		'Truth' Breast cancer present	Breast cancer absent	Totals
Mammography result	Positive	66	8	74
	Negative	21	144	165
	Totals	87	152	239

Sensitivity = 66/87 = 76%
Specificity = 144/152 = 95%

Positive predictive value = 66/74 = 89%
Negative predictive value = 144/165 = 87%

Prevalence = 87/239 = 36%

Derived from data provided by Winchester et al 1983.

CAGE is a mnemonic for four simple questions. Have you ever felt the need to Cut down the amount that you drink, or are you Annoyed by people who criticise your drinking, or have you felt Guilty about your drinking, or have you ever had an Eye-opener (early morning drink) to drink off a hangover, or to steady your nerves?

In one study in primary care, the prevalence of alcoholism was 4% (King 1986), and in another study in medical and orthopaedic out-patients, the prevalence was 20% (Bush et al 1987). This higher prevalence in the hospital setting is to be expected, since alcoholism is associated with medical (e.g. liver disease, gastrointestinal haemorrhage) and orthopaedic (e.g. alcohol-related trauma) admissions. The sensitivity and specificity of the CAGE questionnaire were similar in the two settings, therefore in Table 13.4 the sensitivity and specificity have been held constant.

The values of the individual cells in Table 13.4 can be deduced if the prevalence, sensitivity and specificity are known. In the primary care population of 1000 people with 4% prevalence, 40 people would be alcoholics. Given that the sensitivity of the CAGE questionnaire is 80%, then 32 (80% of 40) alcoholics would be correctly identified and 8 (40 – 32) would have been missed by the test. If 40 people are alcoholics, then 960 (1000 – 40) are not. With a specificity of 95%, the test will have correctly identified 912 of these (95% of 960), but have mis-identified 48 of them (960 – 912) as being alcoholics when in fact they were not. You can do exactly the same exercise to fill in the cells for the hospital population. Table 13.4 B has been left

Table 13.4 The effect of prevalence on predictive value: the performance of the CAGE questionnaire in a primary care and a hospital population

		'Truth': alcoholism present			'Truth': alcoholism present		
		Yes	No	Totals	Yes	No	Totals
CAGE	Positive	32	48	80			
questionnaire	Negative	8	912	920			
	Totals	40	960	1000	200	800	1000

A. Primary care population
Sensitivity = 80%
Specificity = 95%

B. Hospital population
Sensitivity = 80%
Specificity = 95%

Prevalence = 4%

Prevalence = 20%

Positive predictive value = 32/80 = 40%
Negative predictive value = 912/920 = 99%

Positive predictive value = 80%*
Negative predictive value = 95%*

Notes
In this illustration, answering yes to two or more questions in the CAGE questionnaire has been taken to be a positive result. As will be seen later on in the chapter, different definitions of 'positive' can be used.

*To see how the values for positive and negative predictive values for the hospital population are derived, see page **153**.

Data taken from King (1986) and Bush et al (1987).

blank to allow you to work out what should be in each of the cells. Try it! (The answers are given in the example at the end of the chapter.)

Having filled in all the cells, we can then see that the positive predictive value of the CAGE questionnaire in the primary care population is 40% (32/80). In other words, even if someone in this population is identified as positive by the CAGE questionnaire, it is more likely than not (60% vs 40%) that they are not alcoholics. Conversely, in the hospital population, with a prevalence of 20% alcoholism, someone identified as positive by the CAGE questionnaire has an 80% chance of being a genuine alcoholic.

Therefore, it can be seen that diagnostic tests seem to work better in populations where there is more disease. A positive result in a hospital patient is more likely than not to be a true positive, whereas a positive result in a primary-care patient is more likely than not to be a false positive. This is perhaps one of the explanations for the apparent over-investigation of patients in hospital, and under-investigation of patients by general practitioners. Guidelines for investigations based on hospital populations, or patients referred to specialists will be based upon a population with a high prevalence of disease, and therefore may not translate well to a community-based setting where the prevalence of disease is low. A corollary of the better predictive value of a positive test in hospital is that the negative predictive value of a test will actually be better in the community. If you look back at Table 13.4, you will see that the negative predictive value of the CAGE questionnaire is 95% in the hospital setting and 99% in the community setting. Thus, the chance that someone who screens negative with the CAGE questionnaire is really an alcoholic is 1% (100% − 99%) in the community and 5% (100% − 95%) in hospital – in this situation probably not a clinically important difference.

The measure of test accuracy that is most useful when it comes to interpreting test results for an individual patient is something called the *likelihood ratio*. Unfortunately, while simple to use, these can be more difficult to understand than the traditional measures of test accuracy. Therefore, we will approach likelihood ratios first of all from the point of view of how they are used, and then consider what they actually mean.

2. INTERPRETING RESULTS OF TESTS FOR INDIVIDUAL PATIENTS

We have seen from the discussion above that it can be difficult interpreting a result for an individual patient simply knowing sensitivity and specificity. What the health-care professional needs to know is the predictive value of a test, but since this depends upon the prevalence of disease, which will vary from population to population, this has to be worked out for each different population, or indeed for each individual patient. Within a primary care population, the prevalence of breast cancer will be much lower in women

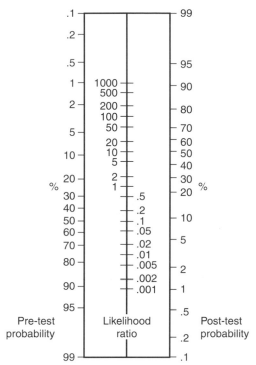

Figure 13.1 A nomogram for applying likelihood ratios (adapted from Fagan 1975 and Sackett et al 1991).

without breast lumps than in women with breast lumps (see above). Thus, the predictive value of the test depends both upon how good the test is, and what is the prevalence of disease in the sort of person to whom the test is being applied. In this context, prevalence can be referred to as *pre-test probability*. Pre-test probability reflects the likelihood that a patient has the disease before you carry out the diagnostic test. Whereas prevalence as a term is applied to populations, pre-test probability is applied to individuals. Essentially, they both mean the same thing when it comes to interpreting diagnostic tests.

Another way of thinking about predictive value is that it reflects the likelihood that a patient has the disease after you have carried out the diagnostic test. This can be referred to as *post-test probability*. Thus, in Table 13.4 in the hospital population, the post-test probability of alcoholism if the test was positive was 80% (= positive predictive value), and the post-test probability of alcoholism if the test was negative was 5% (100% − negative predictive value). When thinking about individual patients, pre-test probability (i.e. probability of disease before you did the test) and post-test probability (i.e. probability of disease after you did the test) are more useful terms than prevalence and predictive value.

So, to apply a diagnostic test to an individual in your practice you need to consider how likely the disease is before you do the test (pre-test probability). Then perform the diagnostic test, and interpret the result not as a simple yes/no answer, but as a probability that the patient has the disease now that you have performed the test (post-test probability). Although this might sound complicated, you are already doing this subconsciously whenever you consider whether a patient has a diagnosis. As we saw when we worked out the contents of the individual cells in Table 13.4, we can derive post-test probabilities using sensitivity and specificity, but it is quite laborious. This is where likelihood ratios come in as a measure of test performance, since, together with a simple nomogram (Fig. 13.1), they can be used to derive the post-test probability from the pre-test probability and the result of the diagnostic test. Like sensitivity and specificity, likelihood ratios do not change as prevalence changes.

Examples of using likelihood ratios to interpret test results

Scenario 13.1

You are a GP. A woman, aged 54, comes to you having just been for a screening mammogram. She has just had a letter to inform her that she needs to be followed up in a specialist out-patient clinic, because the mammogram was abnormal. She wants to know whether or not this means she has breast cancer. You examine her breasts, and find no abnormality. What is the answer to her question?

You estimate the probability that she had breast cancer before the test was performed as being 0.8%. You base this on a paper you came across which evaluated a breast screening programme (Garvican & Littlejohns 1996) – see Table 13.2. You look up the likelihood ratio for a positive test result for mammography, and find it to be 12.6. Using the nomogram, you line up with a ruler a pre-test probability of 0.8% and a likelihood ratio of 12.6, and read off the post-test probability of about 9% (Fig. 13.2). Therefore, you reassure your patient that although the test was positive, it is still unlikely that she has breast cancer, in that only 9 women out of 100 in her situation will actually turn out to have breast cancer.

Scenario 13.2

Another woman, also aged 54, comes to see you. She has recently had a normal mammogram, but is worried because she recently read in a magazine that mammography could miss breast cancer, and wants to know whether

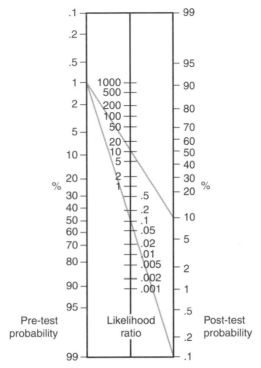

Figure 13.2 Applying a nomogram to interpret possible results of breast cancer screening.

it is possible that she does have breast cancer after all. On examination, her breasts are normal. What is the answer to her question?

You estimate this patient's pre-test probability as being 0.8%. You look up the likelihood ratio for a negative test result for mammography and find it to be 0.13. You use the nomogram again, this time lining up a pre-test probability of 0.8% with a likelihood ratio of 0.13 (Fig. 13.2). You read off a post-test probability of 0.1%. Therefore, you reassure the patient that it is extremely unlikely that she has breast cancer at the moment in that only 1 woman out of 1000 in her situation who has had a normal mammogram really has breast cancer.

As you might have anticipated, you will see that the post-test probability in Scenario 13.1 above is the same as the positive predictive value in Table 13.2, and the post-test probability in Scenario 13.2 is the same as 100% − 99.9%, 99.9% being the negative predictive value shown in Table 13.2.

Estimating pre-test probability

It will have become clear from the examples above that you cannot use a likelihood ratio to interpret a test result for an individual patient without estimating the pre-test probability. You might view this as a weakness of the approach, but it is in fact a strength. The truth of the matter is that you cannot correctly interpret the result of a diagnostic test without considering the pre-test probability, and by using a likelihood ratio, you force yourself to do so.

So how do you estimate a pre-test probability? There are four main sources of information:

- research papers evaluating diagnostic tests
- epidemiological studies and national statistics
- audit data
- clinical experience.

Research papers in which the diagnostic test was evaluated may give valuable information, since it will be possible to derive the prevalence of the disease in the study population. If you think your patient would have been in the study, then you can use the prevalence in the study as your patient's pre-test probability. If not, then you need to decide whether your patient is likely to be at higher or lower risk of the disease than the study patients, and revise the estimate accordingly.

Epidemiological studies and national statistics that look at the incidence and prevalence and risk factors for disease can be used to inform estimates of pre-test probability. It is useful to distinguish between prevalence and incidence here. Prevalence (see above) reflects the number of cases (old and new) in a population at a given point in time. *Incidence* can be defined as the number of new cases in a population over a given period of time. Thus, the prevalence of breast cancer in women aged 50 to 64 is about 8 per 1000 women, whereas the incidence of breast cancer in women aged 50 to 64 is 2.5 per 1000 women per year (Office for National Statistics 1997).

In deriving pre-test probability, both can be useful depending upon the type of disease being tested for. You will need to decide on which is most appropriate depending upon what you are testing for. If you are testing for sudden onset of a new disease, such as say emergency investigation of chest pain to diagnose myocardial infarction, incidence is what is needed. If, on the other hand, you are seeking to diagnose chronic heart failure, then prevalence is likely to be more relevant. If you are considering a diagnosis of cancer, then national statistics may be of some use, since most countries have cancer registration data from which incidence rates for cancer are derived.

Data from epidemiological studies and from national statistics can be useful in estimating pre-test probabilities in healthy patients who are screened for disease, but they are of limited use in estimating pre-test probabilities in patients who present with specific complaints. The incidence of a disease will be much higher in people with symptoms than in people who are symptom-free. Most epidemiological studies will use as their denominator the whole population rather than simply the population with symptoms. For example, in Denmark, which is considered to have a high incidence of inflammatory bowel disease, the incidence of Crohn's disease was found to be 5.4 per 100 000 women per year (Fonager et al 1997). The denominator includes all women. The incidence of Crohn's disease in women with a relevant symptom (e.g. diarrhoea) would be much higher, and it is this incidence that would be relevant for a general practitioner considering whether to request colonoscopy in such a patient. Unfortunately, such data are not usually available.

The pre-test probability should be derived from all the information that the health-care professional has to hand, including the history, clinical examination findings, and any diagnostic tests already carried out. Such an individualised estimation of pre-test probability cannot come from research papers, though it may be informed by them. For example, you might have a lower threshold for doing a chest X-ray in someone who smokes with a persistent cough than a non-smoker with the same symptom. Instead, the health-care professional must rely on local audit data and clinical experience. This may sound a bit of a cop-out for evidence-based health care, but interpretation of diagnostic tests is an area where integration of 'individual clinical expertise with the best available external clinical evidence from systematic research' (Sackett et al 1996) comes into its own. Experienced health-care professionals will intuitively take account of pre-test probability in interpreting diagnostic test results, even if (as is quite likely!) they have never heard of the term, or of likelihood ratios. An attraction of the pre-test probability and likelihood ratio approach to the interpretation of diagnostic tests is that it makes explicit something that has been done implicitly for a long time.

You may be put off by the imprecision of the way in which pre-test probability can be estimated, but it is important to keep things in context. Often, you can be quite a long way off in terms of your pre-test probability, but still come up with the correct interpretation of the test. Going back to the example of mammography and breast cancer, the best estimate of pre-test probability of 0.8% in a middle-aged woman without a palpable breast lump gives a post-test probability of 9% if she has a positive mammogram (i.e. breast cancer unlikely). How high would your estimate of pre-test probability have had to have been, for you to misinterpret this positive result? Well, if we take misinterpreting the test as believing that breast cancer was more likely than not in this patient (i.e. post-test probability of >50%), we can work out using a nomogram what our pre-test estimate of probability would have had to have been. Lining our ruler up against a post-test probability of 50%, and a likelihood ratio of 12.6, we can see that the pre-test probability would need to have been at least 8% (Fig. 13.3). This is a 10-fold over-estimation of the true pre-test probability.

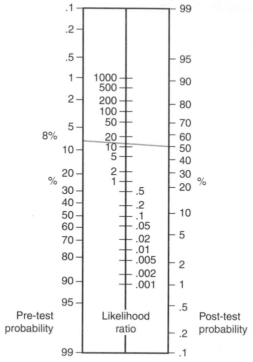

Figure 13.3 Pre-test probability: how wrong do you have to be to get the interpretation of the test result wrong?

What is a likelihood ratio?

So far, while we have shown how to use likelihood ratios to interpret the results of diagnostic tests, we have skirted around saying what a likelihood ratio actually is, and why you need a nomogram to interpret it.

Likelihood ratios come from a mathematical theorem, called Baye's theorem, which states that:

pre-test odds × likelihood ratio = post-test odds.

In other words, if you multiply the pre-test odds of disease by the likelihood ratio of the test, you get the post-test odds of disease. You will see that Baye's theorem is expressed in terms of odds rather than probabilities, which is a little unfortunate because generally speaking we tend to find probabilities easier to understand than odds.

Gamblers amongst you will however be quite familiar with odds. If we say that the odds that a horse will win a race is 1:3, we mean that for every time the horse wins the race, there will be three times that it does not win the race. In other words, the probability that the horse will win the race is actually 1/4, or 25% *not* 1/3!). In the probability of 1/4, the one represents the one time that the horse will win the race and the four represents the three times the horse will not win the race, plus the one time that it will.

The nomogram allows us to use the likelihood ratio while working in probabilities rather than odds. If we did not have a nomogram, we would either have to work in odds (which can be very confusing!), or alternatively, convert our pre-test probability to an odds, then multiply that odds by the likelihood ratio to derive a post-test odds, which we can then convert back to a probability. While this is mathematically reasonably straightforward, as long as you understand the relationship between odds and probability, it is easier to forget all this, and simply use the nomogram!

But what does a likelihood ratio actually mean? Those of you who have done any simple algebra will recognise that the formula for Baye's theorem given above could equally be written as:

$$\text{likelihood ratio} = \frac{\text{post-test odds}}{\text{pre-test odds}}$$

Thus, the *likelihood ratio* is a ratio of the post-test odds to the pre-test odds. Therefore, it reflects how much the odds of disease will change after the test has been carried out. If the likelihood ratio is greater than 1 (i.e. the post-test odds are greater than the pre-test odds – a positive test), then the likelihood of disease after the test is greater than it was before the test. If the likelihood ratio is less than 1 (i.e. the post-test odds are less than the pre-test odds – a negative test), then the likelihood of disease after the test is less than it was before the test. The higher the likelihood ratio for a positive test, the better the test is at diagnosing disease; the lower the likelihood ratio for a negative test, the better the test is at diagnosing non-disease. As a rule of thumb, diagnostic tests with positive likelihood ratios greater than 10 and/or negative likelihood ratios less than 0.1 can be thought of as fairly powerful tests. A likelihood ratio of 10 means, literally, that the odds of disease are 10 times greater than they were before the test was performed. A likelihood ratio of 0.1 means that the odds of disease are one-tenth what they were before the test was performed.

What about tests which do not give yes/no answers?

Of course, many tests do not actually give simple positive or negative answers. There may be borderline results, there may be several categories of result, or indeed, the results may be continuous, e.g. blood glucose. This can be illustrated by going back to the CAGE questionnaire for diagnosing alcoholism. In Table 13.4, two answers of 'yes' to the four questions was taken to indicate a positive result. However, we have lost a lot of information by summarising the data in this way. Among the 'negative' results, someone who answers 'no' to all four questions is less likely to be an alcoholic than someone who answers 'no' to three questions. Similarly, among the 'positive' results, someone who answers 'yes' to all four questions is more likely to be an alcoholic than someone who answers 'yes' to two of the questions. This is shown in Table 13.5, which gives the likelihood ratios for each level of response to the CAGE questionnaire in a study performed in patients attending a general medical clinic (Buchsbaum et al 1991). In this particular population, the pre-test probability of alcoholism was 36%. Using the likelihood ratios in Table 13.5 and the nomogram in Figure 13.1, the post- test probabilities (also shown in Table 13.5) can be derived (try it!). Thus, likelihood ratios can be quoted for any value of a test result, rather than simply reducing it to 'positive' or 'negative'. Using the CAGE question-naire, a 'positive' result of 4/4 is associated with a likelihood ratio of 100, whereas a 'positive' result of 3/4 is associated with a likelihood ratio of 13.

Sometimes, evaluations of diagnostic tests that have multiple or continuous results can be represented as a *receiver operating characteristic (ROC) curve*. This is essentially a graphical representation of what happens to test sensitivity and specificity as the definition of a 'positive' test is changed. For example, there is a screening test for prostate cancer which involves analysis of blood for prostate specific antigen (PSA). PSA is present in the blood in varying amounts in different people, but men with high PSA levels are more likely to have prostate cancer than men with low PSA levels.

An ROC curve for serum PSA in prostate cancer is shown in Figure 13.4 based on data from Morgan et al (1996). The range of possible values of PSA is from 1 to 15. If an 'abnormal' PSA is taken to be relatively low, say 6 or above, then it can be seen from Figure 13.4 that the sensitivity of PSA for prostate cancer would be high (about 94%), but the false positive rate would also be quite high (21%). The *false positive rate* is the proportion of people who do not have prostate cancer who test positive, and is 100% minus the specificity, which is 79% in this case.[2] Conversely, if an 'abnormal' PSA is taken to be high, say 9 or above, the sensitivity of the test has fallen to 68%, the false positive rate has fallen to 10% (and the specificity has risen to 90%). The cut-off that is chosen is a trade-off between sensitivity and specificity. If a low PSA value is taken to be abnormal, then few cases of prostate cancer will be missed, but more people who do not have prostate cancer will have an 'abnormal' test result, and so might worry unnecessarily.

Thus, ROC curves can be a useful graphical way of summarising test performance across the whole range of possible results. They can also be a useful way of comparing the value of different diagnostic tests, or the value of the same test in different groups of people. This is illustrated by Figure

---

[2]Using the nomenclature in Table 13.1, the false positive rate is given by b / (b+d) – the false positives divided by the true negatives plus the false positives.

Table 13.5 Likelihood ratios associated with different responses to the CAGE questionnaire

CAGE score	Likelihood ratio	Post-test probability
0	0.14	7%
1	1.5	45%
2	4.5	72%
3	13	88%
4	100	98%

Data from Buchsbaum et al 1991.

13.5, which shows the ROC curves for three different hypothetical tests: a perfect test, a typical test and a useless test. The better the test, the closer the curve gets to the top left-hand corner of the figure. This can be quantified by calculating the area under the curve. A perfect test will have an area under the curve of 1. A useless test will have an area of 0.5. The better the test, the greater the area under the curve. For example, Morgan et al (1996) found that the PSA test performed better when used in white men (area under the ROC curve: 0.94) than in black men (area under the curve: 0.91). Using an ROC curve to summarise test performance can be particularly useful in meta-analyses of studies of test performance (see Ch. 9).

What if you only know the sensitivity and specificity of the test?

Unfortunately, often studies which are published assessing the accuracy of diagnostic tests do not report likelihood ratios. It is, however, possible to

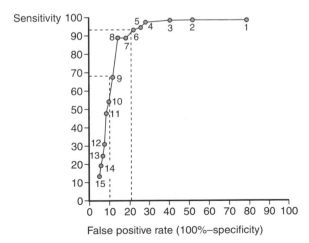

Figure 13.4 ROC curve for PSA values in prostate cancer. Numbers on the graph represent PSA values (adapted from Morgan et al 1996)

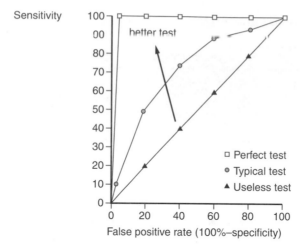

Figure 13.5 Illustrations of different ROC curves.

calculate the likelihood ratios if sensitivity and specificity have been reported.

A likelihood ratio for a positive test result is given by the formula:

$$\text{Likelihood ratio (+ve)} = \frac{\text{sensitivity}}{(100\% - \text{specificity})}$$

A likelihood ratio for a negative test result is given by the formula:

$$\text{Likelihood ratio (-ve)} = \frac{(100\% - \text{sensitivity})}{\text{specificity}}$$

An illustration of these calculations is shown in Table 13.6, using data that was published in a paper assessing the value of an electrocardiogram in identifying heart failure that did not report likelihood ratios (Davie et al 1996).

However, sometimes it can be helpful just knowing sensitivity and specificity if they are very high. Table 13.7 shows data from a study assessing the accuracy of magnetic resonance imaging (MRI) at diagnosing multiple sclerosis (Mushlin et al 1993). In this case, an MRI reading of 'definite multiple sclerosis' has been taken to be a positive result, but all other readings have been counted as negative. Such a cut-off gives a test with

Table 13.6 Calculation of likelihood ratios from sensitivity and specificity

In a study assessing accuracy of electrocardiogram in identifying heart failure, the sensitivity was reported as 94% and the specificity as 61%.

Likelihood ratio (+ve) = 94%/(100% − 61%) = 94/39 = 2.4
Likelihood ratio (−ve) = (100% − 94%)/61% = 6/61 = 0.1

Data from Davie et al 1996.

Table 13.7 Diagnosis of multiple sclerosis by MRI in patients with possible multiple sclerosis – an example of a SpPin

		'Truth' Multiple sclerosis present	Multiple sclerosis not diagnosed	Totals
MRI scan result	Positive Negative Totals	58 105 163	2 138 140	60 243 303

Sensitivity = 58/163 = 36%
Specificity = 138/140 = 99%

Positive predictive value = 58/60 = 97%
Negative predictive value = 138/243 = 57%

Prevalence = 163/303 = 54%

Data from Mushlin et al 1993.

very high specificity, but low sensitivity. You will see that the positive predictive value of such a test is very high. This is a characteristic of tests with high specificity: if the test is positive, it makes the diagnosis very likely. This can be remembered by the mnemonic – SpPin – for a test with high specificity, if the test is positive, then it rules the diagnosis in (Sackett et al 1991).

Table 13.8 shows data from a study assessing the accuracy of a screening test for hearing loss in babies admitted to a special care baby unit (McClelland et al 1992). You can see that in this example, the sensitivity is very high. In this case, the negative predictive value is 100%. In other words, if the test is negative, the diagnosis is very unlikely. This can be

Table 13.8 Screening for hearing loss on a special care baby unit using auditory brainstem evoked potential testing – an example of a SnNout

		'Truth' Baby is deaf	Baby is not deaf	Totals
Screening result	Positive Negative Totals	36 0 36	44 319 363	80 319 399

Sensitivity = 36/36 = 100%
Specificity = 319/363 = 88%

Positive predictive value = 36/80 = 45%
Negative predictive value = 319/319 = 100%

Prevalence = 36/399 = 9%

Data from McClelland et al 1992.

remembered by the mnemonic – SnNout – for a test with high sensitivity, if the test is negative, then it rules **out** the diagnosis (Sackett et al 1991).

ARE THE RESULTS RELEVANT TO YOUR PATIENT?

So far, we have considered how to interpret results of tests for your patients. However, it may be that you feel that the results of studies done to assess the accuracy of the test are not generalisable (or relevant) to your setting, or you may consider that it would not be helpful to your patient to perform the test.

Generalisability to your setting

One aspect to consider is whether the assessments that have been carried out of test validity are applicable to your setting. We have already seen how predictive value is dependent upon prevalence, so the predictive value of a test in one setting is usually not relevant to another setting. Sensitivity and specificity (and likelihood ratios) are not dependent on prevalence, but they can vary according to the type of patients in which the test is carried out. This variation is referred to as *spectrum bias*. The sensitivity of a test will depend upon the severity of disease in the population being tested. The more advanced or severe the disease, the more likely the test is to identify it. For example, in an evaluation of the accuracy of a dipstick test for urinary tract infection, the test was assessed in two groups: one group in whom the clinician thought that the diagnosis of urinary tract infection was likely on the basis of the clinician's assessment of the presenting symptoms and signs, and one group in which the clinician thought the diagnosis was unlikely (Lachs et al 1992). Not surprisingly, the sensitivity of the dipstick test for urinary tract infection was found to be much higher in the first group than in the second group (92% vs 56%). The first group had more prominent symptoms and signs of urinary tract infection, which reflected more established infection which the dipstick test could identify more easily.

The specificity of a test will depend upon the prevalence of other diseases in the population which might lead to false positive results. The more that other diseases are present, the more likely a false positive result. This was also illustrated in the study which evaluated the dipstick test. In the first group, the investigators found that the specificity of the test was lower than in the second group (42% vs 78%). Again, this is to be anticipated since the more symptomatic group will have a higher prevalence of other diseases which might lead to false positive dipstick tests.

A second aspect to consider is whether the test is carried out the same way in your setting as it was in the study. Some diagnostic tests depend upon the skill of the person carrying out the test, and the skill of the people interpreting the test result. Tests may be carried out in different ways, and it is important to know that it is carried out the same way in your local hospital or laboratory as it was in the study which evaluated the test.

Will it help your patient?

One way to think about whether or not to perform the test is whether it will influence the management of the patient or groups of patients you are likely to see. If you think that a disease is unlikely in a particular patient, it may be that if you carried out the test and it was positive, you would still think that the disease was unlikely, so it would not influence your management. Conversely, if you think that a disease is likely in a given patient, it may be that a negative test result would not stop you treating the patient, since you would still think that the disease is likely whatever the test result. Putting this in terms of pre- and post-test probabilities, in the first instance the pre-test probability of disease is so low, that even with a positive test result, the post-test probability will be less than 50%. In the second instance, the pre-test probability of disease is so high that even with a negative test result, the post-test probability will be more than 50%.

These ideas are illustrated in Figure 13.6, which shows possible diagnosis and treatment thresholds in terms of pre-test probability. What you decide is a 'low' or a 'high' pre-test probability will depend upon the nature of the disease being considered and the treatment offered. For breast cancer, the consequences of missing the disease are potentially very serious. Therefore we screen women with a pre-test probability of breast cancer of 0.8% (see p.140), i.e. in effect we classify this risk as 'intermediate'. At the other end of the spectrum, if the treatment is minor (e.g. aspirin to prevent stroke in someone who has had a transient ischaemic attack), we may initiate treatment with a relatively low pre-test probability, whereas if the treatment is major (e.g. radiotherapy for cancer), we would want a very high probability that the diagnosis was correct before we started treatment.

In practice, knowledge about the accuracy of diagnostic tests will perhaps be most useful when planning protocols or guidelines to manage particular groups of patients. For example, the most accurate way of diagnosing heart failure would be to use an echocardiogram. However, in general practice it

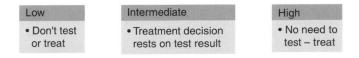

Pre-test probability of disease

Figure 13.6 Thresholds for diagnosis and treatment based on probability that patient has disease (adapted from Sackett et al 1991).

may not be feasible, or indeed a good use of scarce resources, to refer all patients for this investigation with non-specific symptoms such as ankle swelling. There is a 10-fold reduction in the odds of heart failure if the patient has a normal electrocardiogram (ECG) – see Table 13.6 (Davie et al 1996). Therefore, a sensible protocol might include screening such patients with an ECG first. Only those patients with an abnormal ECG would be referred for an echocardiogram.

Any decision about carrying out a diagnostic test will be informed by four major inputs (Fig. 13.7). Not only does knowledge about the patient's symptoms and signs (which informs our assessment of pre-test probability), and our knowledge (preferably in terms of likelihood ratios) about how good the test is influence the decision, but also external factors, such as availability of the test and its cost, and the patient's perspective. The latter is particularly important. For example, one of the antenatal tests that is available for pregnant women is a blood test to screen for Down's syndrome called the triple test. If the test is positive, then the mother would be offered an amniocentesis, which carries a small (1%) risk of miscarriage, to establish whether or not the baby really had Down's syndrome. If the baby did have Down's syndrome, then the mother would be offered a termination. Whether or not it is sensible to have the test depends upon the mother's attitude to having a child with Down's syndrome, her attitude to having a termination and her attitude to the possibility that an amniocentesis will induce a miscarriage of a normal baby. Different women are going to reach different conclusions, according to the value that they attach to the different possible outcomes.

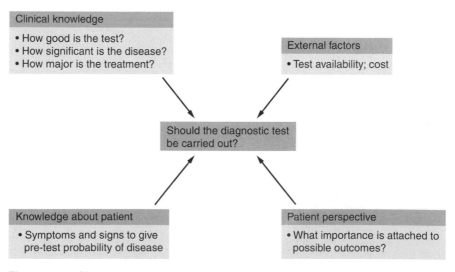

Figure 13.7   Clinical decision-making: diagnosis.

CONCLUSION

An evidence-based approach to deciding whether a test is effective for your patient involves the following steps:

1. Frame the clinical question (see Ch. 2).
2. Search for evidence concerning the accuracy of the test (see Ch. 3).
3. Assess the methods used to determine the accuracy of the test (see Ch. 6).
4. Find out the likelihood ratios for the test.
5. Estimate the pre-test probability of disease in your patient.
6. Apply the likelihood ratios to this pre-test probability using the nomogram to determine what the post-test probability would be for different possible test results.
7. Decide whether or not to perform the test on the basis of your assessment of whether it will influence the care of the patient, and the patient's attitude to different possible outcomes.

WORKED EXAMPLES

Worked example 13.1

If the prevalence of alcoholism is 20% in hospital in-patients, what might one expect the predictive value of the CAGE questionnaire to be, given that it has a sensitivity of 80% and a specificity of 95%? (see Table 13.4)

This is a relevant question, because it allows us to consider how a test evaluated in one population might perform in another population, if we assume that there is no 'spectrum bias' (see p. **150**).

It is possible to construct a two-by-two table comparing test performance against the 'truth' if one knows the sensitivity and specificity of the test and the prevalence of the disease. From this, the predictive value can be calculated.

In this example, if we take a population of 1000 patients:

Step 1. Knowing that the prevalence of disease is 20%, then 20% of 1000 patients, i.e. 200, will have the disease. This means that $1000 - 200$ (i.e. 800) patients will not have the disease. We can therefore fill in the column totals of our two-by-two table:

		'Truth' Alcoholism present	Alcoholism absent	Totals
CAGE	Positive	a	b	
Questionnaire	Negative	c	d	
	Totals	200	800	1000

Step 2. The sensitivity of 80% means that 80% of the 200 people who have the disease, i.e. 160, will be correctly identified by the CAGE questionnaire as having alcoholism. This can be entered into cell 'a'. If 160/200 were correctly identified, this means that 40/200 will have been incorrectly identified as 'negative' on the CAGE questionnaire. This can be entered into cell 'c':

		'Truth' Alcoholism present	Alcoholism absent	Totals
CAGE	Positive	160	b	
Questionnaire	Negative	40	d	
	Totals	200	800	1000

Step 3. The specificity of 95% means that 95% of the 800 people (i.e. 760) who are not alcoholic will be correctly identified as such by the test. 760 can be entered into cell 'd'. If 760/800 were correctly labelled, this means that 40/800 were incorrectly labelled as alcoholic. Therefore, 40 can be entered into cell 'b':

		'Truth' Alcoholism present	Alcoholism absent	Totals
CAGE	Positive	160 (a)	40 (b)	
Questionnaire	Negative	40 (c)	760 (d)	
	Totals	200	800	1000

Step 4. Now that the two-by-two table is complete, the positive and negative predictive values can be calculated:

Positive predictive value = $a/(a + b)$ = $160/(160 + 40)$ = 80%
Negative predictive value = $d/(c + d)$ = $760/(760 + 40)$ = 95%

Worked example 13.2

In a study of the accuracy of clinical assessment of deep-vein thrombosis in patients with suspected DVT, the results of clinical assessment were compared to results of a reference standard investigation, venography:

	Venography result		
	Positive (%)	Negative (%)	**Totals**
Clinical assessment			
High probability of DVT	72 (85)	13	**85**
Moderate probability of DVT	47 (33)	96	**143**
Low probability of DVT	16 (5)	285	**301**
Totals	**135 (26)**	**394**	**529**

Adapted from Wells et al (1995).

A. What is the pre-test probability of a DVT in this population before they are clinically assessed?

This is the same as the prevalence of DVT in the population of patients with suspected DVT, i.e. $135/529 = 26\%$.

B. What is the likelihood ratio for clinical assessment of high probability of DVT?

Likelihood ratio (+ve) = sensitivity / (1 – specificity).

Sensitivity is the proportion of people with DVT correctly identified by the test. This is $72/135 = 53.3\%$ (or 0.533).

Specificity is the proportion of people without DVT correctly identified as 'test negatives'. This is $(394 - 13)/394 = 96.7\%$ (or 0.967).

Therefore, likelihood ratio = $0.533/(1 - 0.967) = 0.533/0.033 = 16.15$.

An alternative method of calculating the likelihood ratio is given in F. below.

C. What is the probability of a DVT in a patient who has been assessed as having a high probability of a DVT (i.e. the post-test probability)?

This can be approached in different ways. The post-test probability is the same as the positive predictive value, which is the proportion of people who test positive who actually have disease. In this case, this is the proportion of people assessed as having a high probability of DVT who have a positive venogram, which is $72/85 = 85\%$.

Alternatively, knowing that the pre-test probability is 26% (see a.), and the likelihood ratio for a positive result is 16.15, then the post-test probability can be read off using the nomogram in Figure 13.1.

Alternatively, knowing that the pre-test probability is 0.26, the pre-test odds of disease are $0.26:(1 - 0.26) = 0.26:0.74 = 0.26/0.74:1 = 0.35:1$. Therefore, the post-test odds of disease are $0.35 \times 16.15:1 = 5.65:1$. This is the same as a post-test probability of $5.65/(1 + 5.65) = 5.65/6.65 = 0.85$.

D. What is the likelihood ratio for clinical assessment of low probability of DVT?

In the chapter, likelihood ratio (–ve) was given as: (1 – sensitivity)/specificity. This is correct where the test gives a positive or negative answer. However, where, as in this case, the test gives a graded, non-dichotomous answer, then you have to be careful how you use this formula.

In essence, clinical assessment of low probability is a 'negative' result. The specificity is given by the proportion of people who had a negative venogram who were identified as having a low probability of a DVT. This is 285/394 = 72.3%, or 0.723.

A 'positive' clinical assessment in this context is moderate or high probability of a DVT. Therefore, the correct sensitivity for this calculation is (72 + 47)/135 = 88.1%, or 0.881.

Therefore, the likelihood ratio = (1 − 0.881)/0.723 = 0.16.

E. What is the probability of a DVT in someone who has been assessed as having a low probability of a DVT (i.e. the post-test probability)?

As with C. above, this can be calculated in different ways. You can apply the likelihood ratio of 0.16 to the pre-test probability of 26% using the nomogram (Fig. 13.1). Alternatively, you can calculate the positive predictive value of a 'negative' result. This is 16/301, i.e. 5%.

F. What is the likelihood ratio associated with a clinical assessment of a moderate probability of DVT?

It is more difficult with this question (though possible) to calculate what the likelihood ratio is in terms of a formula comprising sensitivity and specificity. We think of sensitivity and specificity in terms of two-by-two tables, and in this example, we have three levels of test result (high, moderate or low). We simplified things above by considering the test result as high versus moderate/low (for B.) and low versus moderate/high (for D.). It is easier, when calculating likelihood ratios for more than two levels of test result, to use an alternative definition of a likelihood ratio, which is:

For a given level of a diagnostic test result, the likelihood ratio = proportion of total patients with disease who have given level result divided by proportion of total patients without disease who have given level result.

In this example, the 'given level' is 'moderate probability'. The total number of patients with disease is 135, and the total number of patients without disease is 394. The proportion of total patients with disease who have clinical assessment of 'moderate probability' is 47/135 (0.348), and the proportion of total patients without disease assessed as having 'moderate probability' is 96/394 (0.244).

Therefore, the likelihood ratio = 0.348/0.244 = 1.4.

NB. The likelihood ratios for high and low probability clinical assessments could have been calculated in the same way:

For given level as *high* probability:
Proportion of total with disease = 72/135 = 0.533
Proportion of total without disease = 13/394 = 0.033
Likelihood ratio = 0.533/0.033 = 16.15.

For given level as *low* probability:
Proportion of total with disease = 16/135 = 0.119
Proportion of total with disease = 285/394 = 0.723
Likelihood ratio = 0.119/0.723 = 0.16.

REFERENCES

Buchsbaum D G, Buchanan R G, Centor R M, Schnoll S H, Lawton M J 1991 Screening for alcohol abuse using CAGE scores and likelihood ratios. Annals of Internal Medicine 115:774–777

Bush B, Shaw S, Cleary P, Delbanco T L, Aronson M D 1987 Screening for alcohol abuse using the CAGE questionnaire. American Journal of Medicine 82:321–335

Davie A P, Francies C M, Love M P et al 1996 Value of the electrocardiogram in identifying heart failure due to left ventricular systolic dysfunction. British Medical Journal 312:222

Fagan T J 1975 Nomogram for Baye's theorem. New England Journal of Medicine 293:257

Fonager K, Sorensen H T, Olsen J 1997 Change in incidence of Crohn's disease and ulcerative colitis in Denmark. A study based on the National Registry of Patients, 1981–92. International Journal of Epidemiology 26:1003–1008

Garvican L, Littlejohns P 1996 An evaluation of the prevalent round of the breast screening programme in South East Thames, 1988–1993: achievement of quality standards and population impact. Journal of Medical Screening 3:123–128

King M 1986 At risk drinking among general practice attenders: validation of the CAGE questionnaire. Psychological Medicine 16:213–217

Lachs M S, Nachamkin I, Edelstein P H, Goldman J, Feinstein A R, Schwartz J S 1992 Spectrum bias in the evaluation of diagnostic tests: lessons from the rapid dipstick test for urinary tract infection. Annals of Internal Medicine 117:135–140

McClelland R J, Watson D R, Lawless V et al 1992 Reliability and effectiveness of screening for hearing loss in high risk neonates. British Medical Journal 304:806–809

Morgan T O, Jacobsen S J, McCarthy W F et al 1996 Age-specific reference ranges for serum prostate specific antigen in black men. New England Journal of Medicine 335:304–310

Mushlin A I, Detsky A S, Phelps C E et al 1993 The accuracy of magnetic resonance imaging in patients with suspected multiple sclerosis. Journal of the American Medical Association 269:3146–3151

Office for National Statistics 1997 Cancer statistics: registrations 1990 Series MBI no. 23. The Stationery Office, London

Sackett D L, Haynes R B, Guyatt G H, Tugwell P 1991 Clinical epidemiology, 2nd edn, Little, Brown, Boston

Sackett D L, Rosenberg W M C, Muir Gray J A, Haynes R B, Richardson W S 1996 Evidence based medicine: what it is and what it isn't. British Medical Journal 312:71–72

Wells P S, Hirsh J, Anderson D R et al 1995 Accuracy of clinical assessment of deep-vein thrombosis. Lancet 345:1326–1330

Winchester D P, Sener S, Immerman S, Blum M 1983 A systematic approach to the evaluation and management of breast masses. Cancer 51:2535–2539

14

Is this therapy effective?

Martin Dawes

INTRODUCTION

The aim of this chapter is to enable you to consider one or more treatments and to evaluate in a consistent way their effectiveness in reducing or preventing disease. You will find it helpful to practise these methods and I have included exercises at the end of the chapter for this purpose.

Clinical effectiveness of any procedure or intervention is directly related to the number of people who gain improvement from that procedure as well as how much they gain. It is therefore necessary to examine in detail the results of any controlled trail. The results are often presented in a way that does not make it easy for the reader to understand. This section will enable you to take information from papers and convert bare facts into more meaningful and clinically useful information.

Health-care professionals are continually being informed about details of 'effective' new treatments. This may come from, among other sources, the lay press, medical companies, educational meetings or patients. The difficulty is deciding whether the treatment is likely to be clinically effective (or harmful) in our patients. Effective is itself an emotive word implying some strong property. An important question to ask is 'What is meant by effective?' Is the condition cured while the patient suffers severe side effects or is the pain relieved but the condition deteriorates?

Sometimes a new treatment is so obviously effective that there is no difficulty in making that decision. An example of this is the use of a new anaesthetic gas. On 16 October, 1846, William T.G. Morton demonstrated in public the value of ether for surgery at Massachusetts General Hospital.

Dr Fraser, who had witnessed this demonstration, left Boston on 1 December, 1846, in a wooden paddle steamer. He arrived in Liverpool and reached his mother in Dumfries, Scotland, on 17 December. Two days later, his surgical friends Drs M'Lauchlan and Scott administered ether to a patient there in Dumfries. That same Royal Mail steamer, Acadia, carried a letter and the Boston Daily Advertiser story to Dr Boott at Gower Street, London. Robinson etherised Dr Boott's niece for a molar extraction on 19 December, 1846.

By the end of the year, ether was being used throughout Europe. This history indicates that sometimes if a medication is dramatically effective for frequent serious conditions, little needs to be done about publication as it will become general knowledge very quickly. However, streptokinase (alone or in association with aspirin) is a clinically very effective treatment for acute myocardial infarction producing an important improvement in survival if used soon after the onset of symptoms. Only 20 patients need to be treated to save one life (Midgette et al 1990). It took many years before this important discovery was put into everyday practice (Fibrinolytic Therapy Trialists' (FTT) Collaborative Group 1994). Identifying whether the proposed new treatment is really effective is central to good care. Evaluation of the evidence within clinical research papers describing these therapies is part of that process.

In any clinical therapeutic study there are three explanations for the observed effect:

1. The effect of the treatment
2. Chance variation between the two groups
3. Bias.

Good research will explicitly endeavour to reduce the effects of chance and bias by using special designs.

NATURAL HISTORY OF A DISEASE

Many factors can affect the course and severity of a disease in an individual. We may underestimate anxiety provoked by the fear of illness and similarly the impact of reassurance on this anxiety. Treatment is not just the pharmacological impact of the drug. The knowledge of the diagnosis may be all that is needed to alleviate symptoms. In Box 14.1 I have listed a number of items that may affect the efficacy of a treatment.

Box 14.1   Factors that may affect efficacy of treatment

- Age at diagnosis
- Duration of treatment
- Employment
- Explanation about treatment
- Explanation of disease
- Fear of diagnosis
- Health of family
- Knowledge about diagnosis
- Knowledge of expected outcomes
- Knowledge of side effects
- Pharmacological efficacy of the treatment
- Previous history of disease
- Social aspects
- State of family relationships

The information we give to patients when starting treatment may be critical to the effectiveness of that treatment. The background of the patient including the social and medical history is also relevant. These factors must be taken into account when considering an article describing the effectiveness of any new treatment.

PLACEBO EFFECT

Placebo treatment is effective in its own right and may also have side effects (Editorial 1972). The effect of placebos has been known for centuries. Doctors and quacks have used the impact of the placebo to great effect. The average relief rate from a placebo may be as high as 35% (Beecher 1950). That means that over one-third of patients with certain conditions may get better if you give them all a placebo!

The improvement seen when treating a group with an experimental drug might be due to the placebo effect and not the constituents of that drug. The controlled study will account for this effect by giving a placebo or an experimental drug to the patients.

It is important that the two groups (placebo (or control) and experimental) are similar in all relevant characteristics. Otherwise any difference in treatment effect may not be due to chance or the drug but some other characteristic of the placebo group that differs from the experimental treatment group. For example, the treatment group may have been younger and therefore more likely to recover spontaneously. This difference between the treatment and placebo group is one type of bias.

BASIC DESIGNS OF CLINICAL TRIALS

The discovery of the effect a drug has may occur by chance or design. Once safety and pharmacological tests about dosage have been performed, the drug will be tested on volunteer patients. The randomised control trial is regarded by many as the cornerstone of research design in evaluating the therapeutic effectiveness of a new therapy. Two groups of patients are compared before and after treatment. They are randomly allocated either to one of two experimental drugs or to an experimental drug and a placebo. The placebo drug should be similar in shape, size and colour and have no effect on the problem being treated.

Sometimes patients are given the placebo and the experimental treatments being studied, one following the other. By using the same patients in control and treatment groups you eliminate bias that arises from differences between patients and the design has several statistical advantages. This is called a 'cross-over design'. Occasionally studies will not allocate patients to control or placebo groups. This is usually in diseases where the outcome without treatment is commonly or always fatal.

This raises the issue of 'intention to treat'. How do we know a drug is going to be suitable for all patients? An analysis of the clinical effectiveness of a drug can be applied in several ways. The first is an 'intention to treat' analysis. In this method all patients started on the drug are considered as having taken the drug. Those who stopped because of side effects or did not finish treatment for other reasons are then included in the analysis as treatment failures. In comparison, some analyses will only examine those patients who completed treatment regimens. The latter form of analysis is likely to show a larger benefit of the treatment than the first method. It is important to examine the results section of the article to identify which type of analysis is presented.

DID THE TREATMENT WORK?

After bias has been excluded as much as possible, there are two reasons for a difference occurring between the two groups. The drug may be causing the effect or the effect may be occurring by chance. How does one assess this when reading the article? Normally an article should describe the statistical test used to determine whether the difference occurred by chance. Frequently a paper will describe a difference and then add a p value. These p values are to be found liberally sprinkled through most quantitative research articles. It shows the probability of getting a result as, or more, extreme than the one observed if the difference was entirely due to chance alone. This calculation of p is therefore of great importance in evaluating whether chance is responsible for the observed difference. By excluding chance and bias you are left with the last explanation – that is that the drug was responsible.

WHAT DO WE MEAN BY AND HOW DO WE DESCRIBE RISK?

In everyday conversation we use many terms to describe the risk of an event: risk, chance, danger, gamble, hazard, jeopardy, peril, possibility, uncertainty and venture. We use these terms with adjectives in front of them: high risk, great peril, small chance and little possibility. These phrases are used very commonly and show how accustomed we are to estimating the chances of events occurring in everyday life. What we are not used to is quantifying these chances in any uniform way. We often express chances using comparisons to common or rare events. Winning the lottery was described as less likely than being struck by lightning. In the UK National Lottery six numbers are drawn at random from the set of integers between 1 and 49, which means there are 13 983 816 combinations (the draw order does not matter). This means that the jackpot chance is approximately 1 in 14 million.

Lightning kills 100 people each year in the USA. This is approximately 1 death per 2.5 million people. This is what we accept as an uncommon or rare event. We are not used to talking about percentage probabilities and do not relate well to these terms. The risk of lightning killing a US citizen is 0.00004% probability $((1/2\,500\,000) \times 100$ per annum).

The risk of a 40-year-old, non-smoking male with no previous history of heart disease, normal blood pressure, normal cholesterol, and not diabetic, developing coronary heart disease (CHD) over the next 10 years is 2% (Anderson et al 1991). Another way of expressing this is to say that 2 out of 100 men with the same characteristics will develop CHD. This still may not be high enough for the man to worry about unduly.

We respond to risk depending on our appreciation of the impact of the event. For a 20-year-old man, death is a remote event not necessarily feared greatly. An 85-year-old man may be more likely to appreciate the risk of a fatal event more keenly but it will still depend on individuals as to how they rate their risk. The outcome is the same but the fear, and therefore the reaction to risk of death or disease, varies from individual to individual. This applies to people reading articles. The young researcher reading an article about fractured hips will feel that it is a remote possibility and therefore a large reduction in events would be needed before the researcher felt that the treatment was effective. An older person may feel that, as the personal risk is quite high a smaller benefit of treatment is needed before treatment is clinically effective. This awareness to individual appreciation of risk in specific contexts is important when discussing results with others. Instead of using risk or the reduction of risk to describe the effectiveness of a therapy, an alternative approach may be used.

NUMBERS NEEDED TO TREAT (NNT)

We are often faced with extremely ambitious claims by authors of research on the effect of the intervention. This may be due to the fact that the intervention is indeed very effective. However, the authors will have invested a lot of time in the research and will want to emphasise positive results. Once the effect has been established statistically they will often feel that this is also clinically significant. Unfortunately this is not always the case. The authors will want to put forward the best possible arguments for the use of their intervention and so may use figures that help their argument while omitting figures that are perhaps not so favourable.

The most common approach is to describe the effect of a drug in terms of the risk reduction. The risk is usually of continuing to have, for example, pain or an event such as a stroke or heart attack.

When evaluating an article on a therapeutic manoeuvre it is possible to establish its clinical effectiveness by determining the proportion of patients receiving treatment who gain benefit. At this stage it is useful to consider an example. Alendronate sodium is a relatively new drug that is used in patients with osteoporosis to prevent fractures. As a general practitioner you receive an advertisement from the company containing a section titled 'proof', which states:

The Fracture Intervention Trial was a study, conducted in 11 centres in the USA, of 2027 post-menopausal women aged 55 to 80 years, with hip bone mass density $\leq=0.68$ g/cm^2 and with X-ray evidence of previous vertebral fracture. The reduction in hip fracture was 49%.

At this stage you can do two things: believe the advertising literature or want to check the promotional data for yourself. You request a copy of the paper from a pharmaceutical representative (Black et al 1996). You are happy with the quality of the study (Ch. 5) and now want to determine for yourself the clinical effectiveness. Already you know that there is a 49% reduction in hip fracture. Hip fractures are something that you are keen to prevent as they are associated both with mortality as well as serious morbidity.

From the paper the results in Table 14.1 are drawn. From Table 14.1 it can be seen that there were a total of 33 hip fractures: 22 occurred in the placebo group and 11 in the experimental treatment group. Experimental treatment should reduce the risk of having the fracture.

22 out of 1005 treated with placebo had a hip fracture. This may be presented as a percentage $(22/1005) \times 100 = 2.19\%$. However, in the experimental treatment group there were only 11 fractures in 1022 people (1.08%). These figures may be expressed in the article in the following ways. The relative risk (RR) of having a fracture in the treatment group compared to the control group is calculated by dividing the rate in the treatment group by the rate in the controls (1.08/2.19 = 49%). The relative reduction in risk (RRR) of having a fracture can be calculated by subtracting this relative risk from 100%, or by using the following simple calculation:

$$\frac{CER - EER}{CER} = \frac{2.19 - 1.08}{2.19} = 0.506$$

In this calculation, CER stands for control (placebo) event rate, and EER for experimental event rate. The RRR is expressed as a percentage (51%) and means that the treatment reduced the risk of fracture by 51% relative to that occurring in this control population. You can see already that this

Table 14.1 Results of the treatment of alendronate sodium for preventing hip fracture

	Placebo (control)	Experimental treatment	Total
Hip fracture	22	11	33
No hip fracture	983	1011	1994
Total	1005	1022	2027

Data from Black et al 1996.

statement covers up the fact that the risk itself is 2.19%. Some may think that this is a large risk whereas others may not. As described above, this is a subjective interpretation of risk. How can we use this data and reduce the subjectiveness of the interpretation?

I have shown how the authors may describe the results as a 51% reduction in risk. Let us look at these figures more closely.

The absolute risk is that 2.19% of individuals in the placebo (control) group had a hip fracture. Also that 1.08% of the experimental group had a fracture. The difference (absolute risk reduction or ARR) between these gives us another view of the effectiveness of the treatment. The ARR of this therapy is 1.11% (EER – CER, 2.19 – 1.08).

Another way of considering this is to consider 100 people given this treatment. In this case there would be 1.11 fewer fractures in this group of 100 people compared to a similar group of 100 people who had not received any treatment. Finally, you can see that we are getting near the numbers needed to treat. The numbers needed to treat to prevent 1.11 fractures is 100 people. To calculate how many people we would need to treat to prevent one fracture we calculate the reciprocal of the ARR. In this example 100/1.11 = 90. Therefore to prevent one fracture we need to treat 90 people.

Note. In calculating the ARR it is important to be aware of whether one is working with a percentage or actual numbers. By this I mean that in this example I produced the equation 100/1.11. If I had been using actual numbers instead of percentages, the equation would have been 1/0.0111.

The relative risk reduction for stroke achieved by treating patients with mild-to-moderate hypertension is 50% over 5 years. This means that if I treat patients with mild or moderate hypertension, then I can expect a 50% reduction in stroke compared to the group that does not get treatment. Taken on its own these figures are very impressive and likely to persuade anyone that treatment should be used. It suggests that the treatment is clearly of benefit and should therefore be used. In younger age groups the risk of stroke on treatment is 0.552% (0.00552), over 5 years, compared with a risk without treatment of 1.2% (0.012). These rates are very low. The actual risk reduction is 0.012 – 0.00552 = 0.00648. The reciprocal of this is 1/0.00648 = 154. That means that you would have to treat 154 patients with mild-to-moderate hypertension for 5 years to prevent one stroke.

Some other examples of numbers needed to treat are shown in Table 14.2.

RELATIVE RISK AND ODDS RATIO

What is the difference between relative risk and odds ratio? The answer comes in two parts. You can only calculate the relative risk if you know the baseline or control risk. In a prospective cohort study looking at the effect of smoking that is easy as it is possible to compare the risk of the patients

Table 14.2 Examples of NNTs

Problem	Outcome	Intervention	EER	CER	RRR (CI)	ARR	NNT (CI)
Otitis media	Pain at 2 to 7 days	Antibiotics	10.0%	14.3%	36% (18–50)	4.3%	24
Bell's palsy	Complete recovery	Steroid therapy	77%	68%		9%	11 (6–117)
Acute asthma	Reduce relapse rate	Steroid therapy	8%	16%	58% 21–78)	8%	14 (8–68)

EER, experimental event rate; CER, control event rate; RRR, relative risk reduction; ARR, actual risk reduction; NNT, numbers needed to treat; CI, 95% confidence interval.
For more NNTs, see Bandolier 50th Issue.

who smoke compared with the risk of the non-smokers as shown above. However, prospective cohort studies are expensive and time consuming. It may also involve ethical problems (as in the vaccination example in Ch. 8) to randomly allocate to vaccine or non-vaccine groups for a large trial. If you had performed a case control study as shown in Chapter 8, then your comparison population is not the real population but a matched control group. From Table 8.1 you are unable to calculate the risk of becoming a case in the overall population whether you were vaccinated or not as the study did not measure a population but selected matched controls. The odds of someone having a disease are the number having the disease divided by the number not having the disease. For example 25 out of 100 people have a heart attack, therefore 75 people do not have a heart attack. The odds of having a heart attack in this group of 100 people are $25/75 = 0.33$.

The risk is the number having the event divided by the *total* population. 25 out of 100 people have a heart attack, therefore 75 people do not have a heart attack. The risk of having a heart attack is $25/100 = 0.25$ or 25% As you can see, there is a difference between 0.33 and 25%. When the numbers of the case study get larger, what happens? 25 out of 1000 people have a heart attack, 975 people do not have a heart attack. The odds now are $25/975 = 0.026$ and the risk is $25/1000 = 0.025$. As the event becomes rarer, the odds and the risk become similar.

The point is that in large, well-performed case control studies the odds ratio is similar in meaning to the relative risk. That is if the odds ratio is 3, then you are three times more likely to suffer the event if you have been exposed compared with those who have not been exposed ('exposed' is used to describe not only such things as drugs but also environmental hazards). Similarly, if the relative risk is 3, then you are again three times more likely to suffer. So you can use both odds ratios and relative risk to mean the same thing and most of the time for practical purposes think of them as very similar *but* they are calculated differently, so beware.

PITFALLS IN CALCULATING NUMBERS NEEDED TO TREAT

Clearly it is very important to identify the current numbers from articles. Although the calculation of numbers needed to treat is desirable, many articles do not clearly produce the data in an easily identifiable manner. It is important to have the numbers of all people who were started on treatment and, within those, the number of people who benefited. Some studies report the numbers of patients who benefit without stating clearly how many patients were started in the study.

Let us go back to the article on otitis media (Burke et al 1991). The abstract states that the treatment failure was 14.4% in patients on placebo compared with 1.7% in patients on antibiotics, the odds ratio was 8.21 and the 95% confidence interval was 1.94 to 34.7. Can we determine the numbers needed to treat from this abstract? We also know that 114 received antibiotic and 118 received placebo.

That means that 14.4% of the 118 on placebo were unsuccessfully treated (CER). Similarly, 1.7% of 114 patients were unsuccessfully treated on antibiotic (EER of treatment failure). So from this data we can state that the actual risk reduction (ARR) is $0.144 - 0.017 = 0.127$. Notice how I have converted the data from percentages to actual numbers. This makes the arithmetic easier for calculating NNT. The reciprocal of the ARR is $1/0.127 = 7.87$. By convention we use round numbers to describe NNT and so we would say that the NNT is 8. That is, one would need to treat 8 patients with antibiotics to prevent a 'treatment failure'. Although it is possible to calculate NNT from an abstract, there are drawbacks. We are unable to see clearly what the authors meant by treatment failure. This is critical to our evaluation of the results. In most therapy papers there is data that is not included in the abstract that is necessary for the appraisal of clinical effectiveness.

A word of caution and encouragement. It is not easy to deal with all the arithmetic and it can easily become confusing. It is not the arithmetic that is difficult. It is identifying the correct information to take from the paper. Papers are still not written consistently and this makes it confusing when trying to identify for instance the numbers of patients that benefited from treatment compared to those who did not. Yet you would think that this was the essence of the article and so necessarily should be obvious to the reader. The most frequent confusing factors are identifying how many patients the authors are talking about.

FURTHER ISSUES ON NUMBERS NEEDED TO TREAT

The NNT calculation is being used more and more as a method of assessing clinical effectiveness but still has drawbacks that you should be aware of.

Assuming the quality of the research that generated the NNT is good and that the calculations are appropriate, what other problems exist?

Time of follow-up is critical to your evaluation of the effectiveness of treatment. The example of the treatment of women with osteoporosis is a good example of this. The study was described for a follow-up period of 18 months. What would have happened if you had followed the study for only 6 months or for 36 months? It would be useful to know that the longer you treated women the more benefit you gained as in Figure 14.1.

With the passage of time the actual risk increases. Depending on what happens to the ratio between the placebo or control group and the treatment group, the NNT may also change with time. Where then do you draw the line for a study? Perhaps over 5 years a treatment may have a significantly worse effect than that seen at 2 years.

NNTs are expressed in whole numbers. These numbers can hide a lot of evidence about a treatment. If the NNT was 10 and you were deciding to treat 100 people, does that mean that 90 people will gain no benefit from the treatment? If you are looking at survival then that may be the case. However, if you are looking at the relief of depression, then the answer may be very different. The calculation of the NNT may have used a predetermined threshold for a depression rating score to define depression. The way that these work is that people complete a questionnaire which is scored. This then gives a number above which you may be classed as 'depressed'. The NNT will be useful in determining how many people treated will fall below the threshold. It will not however tell you how many people moved towards normal.

In the treatment of high blood pressure there are several groups of drugs that act in quite different ways. These drugs have been compared. Drug A

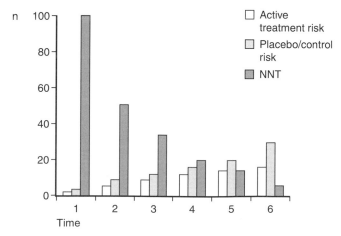

Figure 14.1 NNT and actual risk over time.

will lower blood pressure in a lot of people, whereas drug B may produce the largest fall in blood pressure – but in a smaller number of patients than those receiving drug A. The NNT will only tell you how many achieved a pre-determined improvement, not the total number of people who gained any improvement.

NUMBERS NEEDED TO HARM

Similar equations can be used to identify the number of patients needed to produce harmful side effects from treatment. An example of the need for numbers needed to harm was demonstrated a few years ago. A well-conducted study demonstrated that the risk of developing a deep vein thrombosis (DVT) in the leg while on the oral contraceptive pill was increased in women using more recently developed pills compared with women taking pills developed earlier.

Newspaper articles described this risk as double and the result was that there was a 'pill scare'. This caused anxiety and fear in many women to the extent that there was a rise in unwanted pregnancies brought about by women stopping taking the pill without using an alternative contraceptive.

The risk of developing a DVT on the older pill was 1 per 200 000 years of oral contraceptive use (1:200 000), while the risk on the newer pills was 1:100 000.

The relative risk of developing a DVT on the newer pill was therefore:

$$\frac{\frac{1}{100\ 000}}{\frac{1}{200\ 000}} = \frac{0.00001}{0.000005} = 2$$

So the risk was double. The newspapers were correct in alerting the public that certain pills double your risk – or were they?

The actual increase in risk (ARR) was $0.00001 - 0.000005$. The reciprocal of this is $1/0.000005 = 200\ 000$. This indicates that if you treated 200 000 women for 1 year with newer oral contraceptives, you might expect one additional case of deep vein thrombosis. This information presented at the same time might have had a less alarming impact on the population.

What now follows is some explanation to some of the statistics that you may want to know about. I have tried to stick mainly to the principles of the various statistics you may see in articles discussing therapy. This next section is heavily mathematical so if you do not want to read this section why not move on to the next chapter. It does not include any material required for understanding the rest of the book.

P VALUES

This book is not a statistics textbook but it is worth at this stage just mentioning the importance of statistical significance in research generally. Box 14.2 lists some questions to ask when looking at the statistics of a paper. This checklist will help when checking the statistical quality of the study. There are many things that can go wrong in research, from having too few patients to studying the wrong outcome measure. *P* values are often reported as proof of statistical significance. A convention of stating that *p* is less than a value of 0.05 has been developed. Why is this the case?

Box 14.2   Guidelines for assessing statistics
1. How many patients? (Were there >100 patients?) 2. Was the distribution of the feature normal? 3. What was the size of the effect? 4. Could this have happened by chance? 5. Was $p < 0.05$ or were the confidence intervals separated?

We all have some understanding of probability. A colleague starts tossing a coin repeatedly and it comes up heads every time. At some stage in this process you will start to believe that this result is not just due to chance. If I tossed a coin now and it was heads that would be no surprise. If I do this again and it is still heads you might say 'just chance'. I do it a third time and it is still heads, 'a bit lucky'. I do it a fourth time and it comes down heads. By now, you may say that this is a bit unusual. I do it a fifth time and it is still heads. Do you suspect that something else is going on? Perhaps I am cheating? What this is demonstrating is that we accept things happening by chance until a certain level and then start to suspect that it is not just chance. In most audiences this emergence of disbelief that it is only due to chance appears after the fifth time that the coin is spun and comes up heads. What is happening in this process?

The chance of it being heads on each successive throw is shown in Table 14.3.

It has been demonstrated that when a chance occurrence is expressed in this way we start to disbelieve the phenomenon is purely due to chance at

Table 14.3 Probability of 'heads' being the result of a toss of a coin

Throw	Chance of heads	Probability
1	1/2	50%
2	1/4	25%
3	1/8	12.5%
4	1/16	6.25%
5	1/32	3.125%

the 5% level of probability. This rather vague reason for choosing 0.05 seems very 'unscientific' but at the same time very reassuring to non-statisticians that such an important feature of so many research papers should be based on the concept that this is what we as humans are 'comfortable' with.

When a difference or variation between two measurements occurs we can then describe that difference as being unlikely to have happened by chance. The converse of that is that the difference was due to the mechanism of other factors involved in the study. What it does not prove is that the factors reported by the investigators as being the cause of the variability are necessarily the major cause of that variability; that is, it still might be due to a bias, as opposed to a treatment effect.

The p level is the probability of the difference occurring purely by chance. In other words if p is greater than 5% (0.05), then intuitively we may believe that the difference observed may have occurred by chance and not be due entirely to the intervention.

CONFIDENCE INTERVALS

Some papers use confidence intervals instead of giving a p value. Confidence interval is a way of describing the boundaries between which one is confident that the true measure lies. The confidence intervals for a mean (or average) give us a range of values around the mean where we expect the 'true' (population) mean is located. It reflects both the number of observations and the amount by which each variation differs from the mean. For example, to estimate the mean systolic blood pressure of a general practice adult population, we may take the blood pressure of a random sample of patients, and find that the mean pressure is 136.2 mmHg (95%CI 134.1–138.4). What this means is that we are 'confident' that if we measured the blood pressure of everybody in the practice, we would find that the mean systolic blood pressure was between 134.1 and 138.4. We would be correct 95 times out of 100.

The calculation of confidence intervals is usually based on the assumption that the variable (factor being measured) is normally distributed in the population. The normal distribution curve is essential to much of statistical reasoning.

The normal distribution around a mean (normal curve) was described by Gauss and so is also known as the Gaussian distribution. This curve is symmetrical so that the mean and median (central point of distribution with equal numbers of observations on either side) are the same. The mean is usually labelled μ pronounced 'mew'.

The next characteristic of the normal distribution is the width of the distribution from the mean. This spread is described using the term 'standard deviation' labelled σ (sigma). It is calculated by working out the difference of each measurement from the mean, squaring these differences, dividing the sum of these squared differences by the number of observations, and finally taking the square root:

$$\sigma = \sqrt{\frac{(x - \mu)^2}{n - 1}}$$

where x is the individual observation. (Not a very intuitive calculation!)

As a result of the mathematical proportions of the normal curve it was established that the probability of an observation falling within one standard deviation is 68%, and within two standard deviations 95%. Few physical, biological or social phenomena are entirely normally distributed. However with more than 100 observations, unless the distributions are very odd, this becomes less important in terms of subsequent analysis.

Blood pressure is one of the commonest physiological measurements. This graph shown in Figure 14.2 describes the distribution of blood pressure from a cohort of patients in Oxfordshire recruited at random from general practice.

It shows the normal distribution (line) with the actual distribution behind as a histogram. There were 448 observations. The mean was 136.2, the median 133, the standard deviation 23.5. This means that there was a 68% probability of one of these individuals having a blood pressure between 113 and 160. In this group of people 312 (69%) actually had a blood pressure within that range. Similarly the number of people whose blood pressure was between 89 mmHg and 183 mmHg was 432 (96%). The standard deviation then represents the scatter of the distribution of the individual's blood pressure. The calculation of a confidence interval represents the

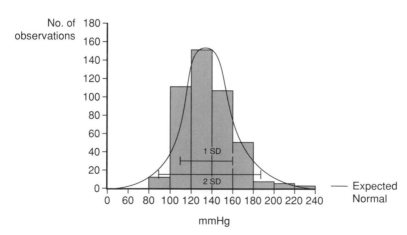

Figure 14.2 Systolic blood pressure in primary care.

likelihood of this mean representing the truth. The more patients the study has, the less wide are the confidence intervals. It also includes within its formula the standard deviation so also reflects the scatter of readings.

In studies looking at the effect of a treatment the results may then contain two means: the measurement on placebo (control) and the measurement on experimental treatment. Each may have a confidence interval in the form of a table or be represented graphically. If the confidence intervals overlap, then you cannot be sure that the difference observed did not occur through chance. More formally, you would usually test whether or not the two means were significantly different from each other by calculating the 95% confidence interval around the difference between the means. If this confidence interval included 0, then you would conclude that the observed difference between the two means might have arisen as a result of chance.

In the blood pressure study the mean of systolic blood pressure in males was 142.3 (95%CI 139.4–145.3) and in females 129.4 mmHg (95%CI 126.4–132.4). The means seem very different and the upper level of the confidence interval for females (132.4) is lower than the lower level of the confidence interval for males (139.4) indicating that the difference is likely to be real.

Another way of displaying this might be a 'box and whisker plot', showing for example the standard error as a box and the confidence interval as a line from top to bottom with the mean in between (Fig. 14.3).

Which is best? *P* values or confidence intervals? *P* values do not give information about the size of the difference between the study groups (Gardner & Altman 1986). Both however do give useful information and authors are now asked to provide both when submitting papers to many journals.

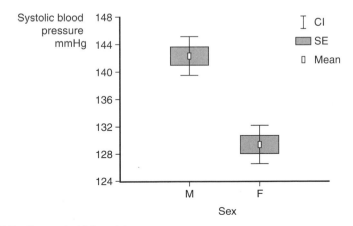

Figure 14.3 Box and whisker plot.

SAMPLE SIZE

The numbers of patients is important in determining the power of a study. Too few patients can lead to two sorts of problems. First, the intervention is shown to be effective when in reality it is not (type I error). One protects against this sort of error by calculating the p value for the results. If the p value is less than 0.05, there is a less than 5% chance that this error has occurred. With small studies, you are less likely to obtain such a p value unless the size of the difference is very large. Second, the study may show the treatment not to be effective when in reality it is (type II error). The larger the sample size, the less likely it is that this error will occur. The methods section of a paper may often specify the risk of committing a type II error. A level of 0.20 for Beta is considered adequate. In other words this would give a 1 in 5 chance of missing a true difference. The statistical power (1-Beta, usually 80%), the Alpha level (0.05, p value) and the difference in outcome (the difference between the two means) are all included in the equation that predicts sample size (Box 14.3).

Box 14.3 Sample size calculation

Prior to using this you must specify the alpha level (usually 0.05 or 5%) and the statistical power, usually 80% (a beta level of 20%).
The equation for a sample size for a comparison of two proportions is:

$$n = \left[\frac{Z_\alpha \sqrt{2\pi_c(1 - \pi_c)} - Z_\beta \sqrt{\pi_t(1 - \pi_t) + \pi_c(1 - \pi_c)}}{\pi_t - \pi_c} \right]^2$$

where n is the number of patients for each treatment group.
Z_α = alpha level
Z_β = power
π_c = Control group proportion developing disease
π_t = Treatment group proportion developing disease

To compare the means from two populations based on a sample of n individuals from each population:

$$n = 2 \left[\frac{(Z_\alpha - Z_\beta)\sigma}{(\mu_1 - \mu_2)} \right]^2$$

σ = standard deviation of the variable of interest
μ = means of the two populations.

CONFIDENCE INTERVALS FOR NUMBERS NEEDED TO TREAT

When reading articles about NNT you will sometimes come across an NNT with a confidence interval (e.g. NNT = 12 [95%CI 8–24]. This is the process for calculating the confidence interval of an NNT. First, you calculate the actual risk of having the undesired outcome (i.e. death) in the group of patients (N^C) taking a placebo (CER) and in those patients (N^E) having the treatment (EER).

Next, you must use some arithmetic. The following equation will calculate the standard error (SE) of the actual risk reduction:

$$SE(ARR) = 1.96 \times \left(\sqrt{\left(\frac{CER \times (1 - CER)}{N^C} + \frac{EER \times (1 - EER)}{N^E} \right)} \right)$$

This standard error is then subtracted and added to the ARR to give limits of standard error on either side of the ARR:

+ve SE = ARR + SE(ARR)
−ve SE = ARR − SE(ARR)

The confidence limits of the NNT are then the reciprocals of the +ve and −ve SEs.

An example may make this clearer. In the otitis media study, treatment failure was seen in 2 out of 114 children in the treatment group. This was in comparison to 17 children out of 118 in the control group.

The CER was 17/118 = 14.4%, while the EER was 2/114 = 1.75%.

SE(ARR) = 1.96 × (√ ((0.144 × (1 − 0.144))/118) + ((0.0175 × (1 − 0.0175))/114
= 1.96 × (√ (0.0011954))
= 1.96 × 0.03457
= 0.0677

ARR = 0.144 − 0.0175 = 0.1265
+ve SE = 0.1265 + 0.0677 = 0.1943
−ve SE = 0.1265 − 0.0677 = 0.0587

NNT = 1/ARR = 7.9
95% Confidence Limits = 1/0.1943 = 5.1 and 1/0.0587 = 17.0

The NNT can be expressed as 7.9 (95%CI = 5.1–17.0). Most confidence intervals have an equal amount of variation between the upper and lower levels. For example, you would have an upper confidence limit of 10 and a lower limit of 6 around a finding of 8, that is 8 (95%CI = 6–10). There is an equal distance between 8 and 10 as there is between 8 and 6. However, in confidence intervals around NNT this is not the case. This is due to the fact that we are really calculating CIs around the ARR and then producing a reciprocal (dividing 1 by the amount). This leads to an unequal distribution.

SUMMARY

After reading all this you may be quite anxious about trying the calculations for yourself. However, like most things in medicine with practice and familiarity, they will become very much easier. The appraisal of a paper describing a therapeutic benefit can appear daunting. The arithmetic is the easy bit. Really! The hard part is getting the numbers out of the paper. So often authors use double negatives or obscure terms when describing the results. You have to search within the tables for the nuggets of information. Papers written more recently are likely to be slightly easier to appraise with information more clearly displayed.

The answer is to practise. Check your results with others. And do not be afraid to have a go. For practice, why not try articles that have been reviewed by Evidence Based Medicine as this journal publishes the NNTs with confidence intervals.

WORKED EXAMPLES

Worked Example 14.1

You are looking after a child with asthma who has to go back into hospital following a recent admission. You wonder whether anything could have been done to prevent this. You contact the information officer of the primary care group and the two of you find and decide to appraise the following article:

Madge P, McColl J, Paton J 1997 Impact of a nurse-led home management training programme in children admitted to hospital with acute asthma: a randomised controlled study, Thorax: 52: 223–228. Reproduced with permission from the BMJ Publishing Group.

Background

Re-admissions to hospital in childhood asthma are common with studies reporting that 25% or more of children will be re-admitted within a year. There is a need for strategies to reduce re-admissions.

Methods

A prospective randomised control study of an asthma home-management training programme was performed in children aged 2 years or over admitted with acute asthma. 201 children were randomised at admission to either an intervention group (n = 96) which received the teaching programme or a control group (n = 105). A nurse-led teaching programme used the current attack as a model for the management of future attacks and included discussion, written information, subsequent follow-up and telephone advice aimed at developing and reinforcing individualised asthma management plans. Parents were also provided with a course of oral steroids and guidance on when to start them.

Results

The groups were similar in degree of social deprivation, length of stay, number of previous admissions, acute asthma treatment, and asthma treatment at discharge. Subsequent re-admissions were significantly reduced in the intervention group from 24.8% to 8.3% in individual follow-up periods that ranged from 2 to 14 months (chi^2 = 9.63; p = 0.002). This reduction was not accompanied by any increase in subsequent emergency room attendances nor, in the short term, by any increase in urgent community asthma treatment. The intervention group also showed significant reductions in day and night morbidity 3 to 4 weeks after admission to hospital.

Conclusions

A nurse-led asthma home-management training programme administered during a hospital admission can significantly reduce subsequent admissions to hospital for asthma. Acute hospitalisation may be a particularly effective time to deliver home-management training.

Tasks

The article fulfils the quality checklist. You decide to work out from the data presented the NNT to prevent subsequent admission using this home-management training. Try doing this yourself now before looking at the answer (p. **178**)

Worked Example 14.2

Lots of your patients seem to be coming back to you following the diagnosis and treatment of lower respiratory tract infections. You decide to see whether this can be reduced and find the following article:

Macfarlane J, Holmer W, Macfarlane R 1997 Reducing reconsultations for acute lower respiratory tract illness with an information leaflet: a randomized controlled study of patients in primary care. British Journal of General Practice 47 (424): 719–722

Background

General practitioners (GPs) prescribe antibiotics to three-quarters of patients who consult with a lower respiratory tract illness (LRTi). In spite of this management, around one-quarter of patients re-consult for the same symptoms within a month.

Aim

To investigate the impact of providing a simple leaflet regarding the natural history of lower respiratory tract symptoms on re-consultation rates for previously well adults presenting to their GP with an LRTi.

Method

76 GPs studied 1014 previously well adults presenting with an illness defined as an LRTi. Management was left to the GPs' discretion. Half of the patients were randomly allocated to receive an information leaflet at the end of the consultation, blinded from the GP. The end point was re-consultation for the same symptoms within 1 month.

Results

Follow-up data was available for 1006 adults, of whom 182 (18%) re-consulted. Fewer patients who received the leaflet (75/505; 14.9%) returned to the surgery compared with those who did not (107/501; 21.4%; $p = 0.007$). The same benefit was found for the 723 (72%) adults treated initially with antibiotics; 16% (60/369) in the leaflet group returned compared with 23% (81/354) in the no leaflet group ($p = 0.02$).

Conclusion

Informing previously well patients about the natural history of LRTi symptoms is an effective strategy for reducing re-consultations, benefiting the patient and the GP; it is likely to reduce antibiotic prescriptions and future patient consultation habits.

Task

Find out what proportion of patients receiving advice return to surgery compared with those who did not receive advice. Calculate from this the ARR and the NNT. What are the confidence intervals of that NNT?

ANSWERS

Worked Example 14.1

What is surprising is that all the data you need to work out both the NNT and the confidence limits of that NNT are already in the abstract!

This is how I did it:

The EER was 8.3% and CER was 24.8%.

The difficult part is sorting out which is control and which is experimental.
The RRR was 66.3% ((24.8 − 8.3)/24.8)
The ARR was 16.5% (24.8 − 8.3)
The NNT was (1/0.164) = 6
The confidence interval of the ARR was worked out using the equation on
pages **174–175**. The numbers for the two groups were as shown below:
SE(ARR) = 1.96 × ($\sqrt{}$ ((0.083 × (1 − 0.083))/96) + ((0.248 × (1 − 0.248))/105)
= 1.96 × ($\sqrt{}$ (0.00257004))
= 1.96 × 0.05069556
= 0.0993633
+ve SE = 0.164 + 0.0993633 = 0.26364902
−ve SE = 0.164 − 0.0993633 = 0.06492241
NNT confidence intervals were:
1/0.26 = 4 and 1/0.065 = 15
NNT = 6 (95%CI 4–15)
  NB. There are aspects to the intervention that are only available from
reading the whole article. If you felt the NNT was impressive enough you
would now have to examine the methodology of the intervention to ensure
that, not only was the quality of the research good enough, but that the
intervention was itself a practical option in your centre.

Worked Example 14.2

21.4% of patients who had no advice (CER) returned to surgery. 14.9% of
those who had received advice returned to surgery (EER). Therefore the
ARR was 6.5%.
1/ARR = 15.4
NNT = 15 (95%CI 9–57).

REFERENCES

Anderson K, Odell P, Wilson P, Kannel W 1991 Cardiovascular disease risk profiles.
    American Heart Journal 121(1 Pt 2):293–298
Beecher H 1950 The powerful placebo. Journal of the American Medical Association
    159:1602–1606
Black D, Cummings S, Karpf D et al 1996 Randomised trial of effect of alendronate on risk of
    fracture in women with existing vertebral fractures. Fracture Intervention Trial Research
    Group Lancet 348(9041):1535–1541
Burke P, Bain J, Robinson D, Dunleavey J 1991 Acute red ear in children: controlled trial of
    non-antibiotic treatment in general practice. British Medical Journal 303:558–562
Editorial 1972 Drug or placebo? Lancet 2(7768):122–123
Fibrinolytic Therapy Trialists' (FTT) Collaborative Group 1994 Indications for fibrinolytic
    therapy in suspected acute myocardial infarction:collaborative overview of early mortality
    and major morbidity results from all randomised trials of more than 1000 patients. Lancet
    343:311–322

Gardner M, Altman D 1986 Confidence intervals rather than P values: estimation rather than hypothesis testing. British Medical Journal Clinical Research Edition 292(6522):716 750

Macfarlane J, Holmes W, Macfarlane R 1997 Reducing reconsultations for acute lower respiratory tract illness with an information leaflet: a randomized controlled study of patients in primary care. British Journal of General Practice 47(424):719–722

Madge P, McColl J, Paton J 1997 Impact of a nurse-led home management training programme in children admitted to hospital with acute asthma: a randomised controlled study. Thorax 52:223–228

Midgette A S, O'Connor G T, Baron J A, Bell J 1990 Effect of intravenous streptokinase on early mortality in patients with suspected acute myocardial infarction. A meta-analysis by anatomic location of infarction. Annals of Internal Medicine 113:961–968

15

Is the intervention cost-effective?

Alastair Gray

INTRODUCTION

In Chapter 10 we set out some guidelines for good practice in economic evaluation. But why do we have to consider cost-effectiveness in the first place? And how can we use the results of economic evaluations in evidence-based practice? Until recently the movement to improve the evidence base of medical practice has put the major emphasis on establishing the *effectiveness* of interventions: broadly, to ask whether there is evidence that an intervention is better than nothing, and if so, how effective it is and how it compares with alternatives. These are fundamental questions, but knowing that an intervention is effective, or even knowing that it is more effective than any alternative, is not a sufficient basis on which to provide that intervention. Already the availability of effective interventions far exceeds our capacity to purchase them all, and the technological frontier of medical science is constantly being pushed outwards, in turn pushing the potential cost upwards.

In the UK, the proportion of total national income devoted to health care has grown steadily from under 4% in 1960 to over 7% in 1996, and real expenditure per person per year (in 1990 £s) has risen from £196 to £707 over the same period, yet choosing what should and should not be provided has not become any less painful. Similarly, countries which devote higher shares of national income to their health care systems – such as Germany (10.5%) or the USA (15%) – also remain locked in debate over priorities, cost-control and value for money.

These problems are very familiar to economists. Indeed, from an economic perspective health care is not fundamentally different from any other good or service. We live in a world of scarcity – scarce time, scarce space, scarce knowledge and skills – and therefore must constantly make choices about alternative courses of action. Individually, should we have the exterior of the house repainted, or put it off another year and put the money towards a summer holiday? Collectively, should we increase spending on schools or on the health service? Professionally, should we appoint another orthopaedic surgeon or expand the domiciliary chiropody service? If funding for elective surgery is suddenly reduced by 20%, who should be removed from the operating lists first? In all of these situations, we have to make a choice, which involves some comparison of the relative costs and benefits of the alternatives. By adopting the framework of economic evaluation, all we are really doing is making this comparison more explicit. Of course explicitness can be uncomfortable and even threatening. But the advantages of explicitness over hunch and guess work are that (a) all the relevant alternatives can be identified; (b) the viewpoint or perspective from which the choice has been made has to be stated; and (c) some attempt can be made to recognise and measure the uncertainty surrounding the choice (Eddy 1992).

So the starting point for health economics is that we have to make difficult choices concerning health-care resources, and that an explicit weighing of costs and benefits surrounding these choices can lead to a better outcome, in which more health gain is obtained with the available resources.

THE COST-EFFECTIVENESS PLANE

One way of thinking about these choices in health care is by means of a simple diagram called the 'cost-effectiveness plane', which is shown in Figure 15.1.

Imagine that we wish to compare therapy A (e.g. a new drug therapy for dyslipidemia) with therapy B, the existing therapy. Along the horizontal axis we can measure whether the new therapy is more or less effective than the existing therapy, and up and down the vertical axis we can measure whether it is more or less costly. Now clearly we need to have accurate information on costs and on effectiveness in order to locate our new therapy on this diagram, a point we will return to below. But let us assume for the present that we have this information, and that the new therapy

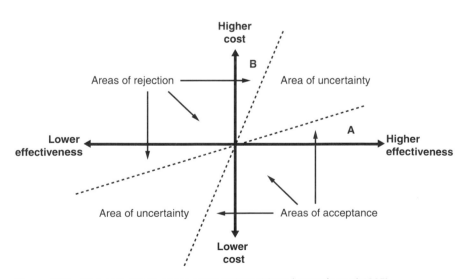

Figure 15.1   The cost-effectiveness plane (adapted from Laupacis et al 1995).

turns out to be more effective than the new therapy and less costly. It will be in Quadrant II (quadrants are numbered clockwise), and we can safely assume that it will be accepted over the existing therapy: it 'dominates' the existing therapy. Conversely, if the new therapy turns out to be less effective and more expensive (Quadrant IV), it will be rejected.

Now let us imagine that the new therapy is a lot more effective and just a little bit more costly: say at point A in Quadrant I. Probably this will still be acceptable, as offering a major health gain for relatively low additional cost. But suppose the new therapy is only fractionally more effective than the existing therapy and is very much more costly: for example, at point B in Quadrant I. Now the balance has probably tipped against the new therapy and it is adjudged to be too expensive in relation to the benefits it offers.

So at what point does acceptability turn to uncertainty and then into rejection? That will depend on many things, including the total resources available and alternative uses of those resources for other health-care interventions. For example, we can easily imagine that a new therapy, which is known to be more effective than the existing alternative and also more costly, could be well under the line of acceptability in the USA, in the uncertainty zone in the UK and well into the rejection zone in Sub-Saharan Africa. So the judgement we reach will depend on the relative effectiveness and costs of the therapy compared to the existing alternative, but also on the resources available.

The simple but powerful logic underlying Figure 15.1 is in essence the cost-effectiveness approach. In fact the *cost-effectiveness ratio* is simply the slope or gradient of a line from the origin to any point in Figure 15.1. This slope is the ratio of cost to effectiveness, and cost-effectiveness can be defined as the ratio of the net difference in costs between two therapies to the net difference in effectiveness. Of course there are many conceptual and empirical difficulties involved in this approach, but it is important to keep hold of the essential simplicity: if we can systematically measure and compare the costs and the effectiveness of health interventions, we can in principle maximise health gain by selecting those which are most cost-effective, then the second best, then the third best, until our budget is exhausted. Any other approach will result in less health gain.

COST-EFFECTIVENESS: AN EXAMPLE

To illustrate the cost-effectiveness approach let us take a recently published economic evaluation and look at it from the point of view of the checklist we set out in Box 10.1 (p.102).

A. The framework
1. *The type of analysis being performed should be clearly stated and justified.*
2. *The background of the problem being addressed, and the general design of the programme under investigation, including the target population, should be stated.*

3. *The comparator programme should be described.*
4. *The perspective and time horizon of the study should be stated.*

Recent large trials have provided convincing evidence that drug therapy to lower cholesterol is effective in reducing fatal and non-fatal coronary events. One such trial, the Scandinavian Simvastatin Survival Study (4S), showed that lowering cholesterol levels with simvastatin reduces mortality and morbidity. These results were obtained in a treatment population consisting of men and women at various ages from 35 to 70 years with angina pectoris or previous acute myocardial infarction and with total cholesterol levels before treatment of between 213 and 309 mg/dl (4S 1994).

However, the premise of health economics is that evidence of effectiveness is not *sufficient* reason to advocate the widespread use of cholesterol-lowering drugs in such patients. The cost per patient per year of such therapy would typically be around £540, and it is possible that up to 8% of all men and women aged 35 to 70 would fit the eligibility criteria of such trials. Treating everyone who might benefit would therefore be very costly: in fact, it could represent more than 20% of the existing total drug budget. So before widespread use is recommended, the cost-effectiveness of cholesterol lowering therapy should be demonstrated.

A search of the literature would identify a large number of published cost-effectiveness analyses of cholesterol-lowering therapy. But most of these are simulations or modelling exercises based on cost and effectiveness data taken from a wide range of different sources. However, an economic evaluation was performed alongside the 4S study, and used cost and effectiveness information from that trial to estimate the cost-effectiveness of simvastatin treatment, defined as the cost per year of life gained with simvastatin therapy compared with placebo (quality of life was not considered) (Johannesson et al 1997).

The perspective adopted by this study included health-care system costs and the lost production costs arising from morbidity from coronary causes. The trial had a follow-up period of 5 years, but from an economic perspective this was not an adequate time horizon, as the differences in survival detected after 5 years might be expected to continue into the future. So increased life expectancy beyond the end of the trial was extrapolated from the information produced within the follow-up period on survival. Note that it is common to have to combine trial results with some modelling in this way, especially if the main outcome is survival (Buxton et al 1997).

B. Data and methods
5. *All resources of interest in the analysis should be clearly identified, measured and valued.*
6. *All outcomes of interest in the analysis should be clearly identified, measured and valued.*

7. *Methods of obtaining estimates of effectiveness, resource use, unit costs and quality-of-life valuations should be given, alongside the sources of information.*

The resources of interest were the drug itself, plus the treatment of coronary events, plus the time off work of patients as a result of a coronary event. The cost of the drug was the official retail price, the cost of health-care resources was based on data from four hospitals with detailed accounting procedures, and the cost of time off work was based on average earnings of full-time workers. As noted above, the outcome was defined in terms of life years gained, and the data for outcomes and resource use were taken directly from the 4444 patients in the trial.

C. Results

8. *The base case results in terms of costs, effectiveness, and incremental cost-effectiveness ratios, and the uncertainty surrounding these, should be clearly set out.*

Table 15.1 summarises the main results of the study. It can be seen that the authors show the cost, years of life gained and then the cost-effectiveness ratio, and not just the ratio itself. They also show separate results for men and women, and separate results for health-care costs alone and when, including work-time lost. Thus for men the cost of the intervention (i.e. the drug and monitoring cost) would be $2242, but this would be offset by $718 in savings from reduced morbidity, so the net cost would be $1524. On average the gain in life expectancy would be 0.28 years, or just over 3 months, so that the cost per life-year gained would be $1524/0.28 = $5400. Adding in the savings resulting from less time off work, the net cost falls to $459 and so the cost-effectiveness ratio falls to $1600 per life-year gained. The authors also present results for different age groups, and for patients with different pre-treatment cholesterol levels.

Finally, the authors present the results of a sensitivity analysis, in which different base case assumptions and values are altered to assess their effect on the results. This analysis is presented graphically in Figure 15.2, with the base case being a 59-year-old woman with a cost per life-year gained of $10 500. Thus, when the reduction in risk obtained from the therapy is set at 20%, the cost-effectiveness rises to $15 300, and when the reduction in risk is set at 34% the cost-effectiveness ratio falls to $7300. Such a sensitivity analysis allows the decision-maker to assess the robustness of the results.

9. *The results should be placed in the context of other relevant economic evaluations.*

In discussing their results, the analysts cited four other cost-effectiveness studies published in the previous 7 years, in the areas of hormone replacement therapy, screening for hypertension and cholesterol-lowering treatment.

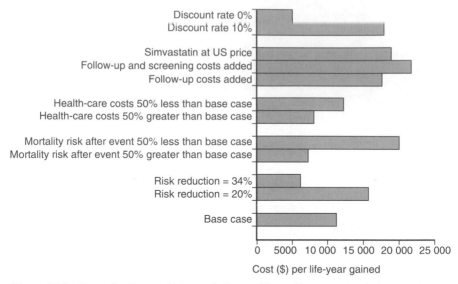

Figure 15.2 Example of a sensitivity analysis cost ($) per life-year gained, simvastatin treatment for 5 years in a 59-year-old woman with coronary heart disease and a pre-treatment total cholesterol level of 261 mg/dl.

D. Discussion

10. The relevance of the study for policy questions, and any ethical or distributive implications, should be discussed.

Based on their analysis, the authors conclude that 'the estimated cost-effectiveness ratios were well within the range that was considered cost-effective in other studies', and therefore that in patients with coronary heart disease, simvastatin therapy is cost-effective among both men and women at the ages and cholesterol levels studied.

Comments on the cost-effectiveness example

To consider this study carefully against the checklist, you would of course have to read the original article in detail. However, it should be fairly clear from the information given above that this is a well-conducted study which in most respects passes the checklist points. There are some points which you may have noticed:

• Some aspects of cost, such as costs incurred by patients in attending clinics, were not included. You may judge that these were unlikely to be important in this instance; but in some studies they could be significant.

• Outcome was measured in term of survival only, and did not include quality of life. This was justified in the article on the grounds that valid weights or valuations for the health states in the study did not exist, but if quality of life was not very good (and remember all patients in this trial had a history of heart disease), then the quality-adjusted life-years (QALYs) added by therapy could be significantly less than the life-years added.

• The costs reported in the article are the average costs prevailing at present. However, often in economic studies we are interested in the effect of a change at the margin, such as reducing length of stay by 1 day, treating more patients with cholesterol-lowering therapy, or extending a dental surgery's opening hours by 3 hours per week. The cost of these changes is the *marginal cost*, which can be defined as the change in total cost divided by the change in total output or quantity.

Suppose a dental practice was currently open from 9 am until 5 pm with total running costs for the premises of £75 000 and total visits of 25 000 annually. Hence the average cost per visit for the premises is £3. Suppose it is now decided to extend surgery hours on 2 nights per week. The total cost goes up to £82 000 and the total number of visits goes up to 26 000, so the average cost has only increased fractionally to £3.15 per visit (82 000/ 26 000). However, if we consider the marginal cost, an additional 1000 visits are costing an additional £7000 per year, so in fact the marginal cost per visit is £7, very much more than the average cost. Indeed, the difference between the average and marginal cost is so great that the practice may decide to review the decision to extend opening hours! Note, however, that marginal costs may also be lower than average cost.

• Marginal cost refers to the consequences of expanding or contracting the size of a specific service or activity: more opening hours in a surgery or fewer beds in a ward. But often the decision is whether to expand the whole scope or coverage of a programme, for example from breast cancer screening for those aged 60 and over to breast cancer screening for those aged 50 and over. The change in cost that occurs when this happens is referred to as the *incremental cost*, and so the change in cost in relation to the change in outcome of such a change would be called the *incremental cost-effectiveness ratio*, or ICER. The results are correctly reported in the article as the incremental cost-effectiveness ratio, that is, the additional costs and effectiveness compared to placebo therapy. However, a decision-maker may wish to consider other increments of therapy. For example, patients could be treated at different doses, each with different cost and effectiveness combinations.

Figure 15.3 shows some results from a different cost-effectiveness analysis of cholesterol-lowering therapy, where patients can be treated at 20 mg, 40 mg or 80 mg per day. To treat a cohort of 65- to 74-year-old men with a 20 mg dose would have a lifetime cost of $3.6 billion, and would save a total of 348 000 life-years, giving a cost of $10 400 per life-year saved. On Figure 15.3 the life-years gained are plotted along the X-axis, the cost along the Y-axis, and the slope of the line to that point is the cost-effectiveness ratio of $10 400.

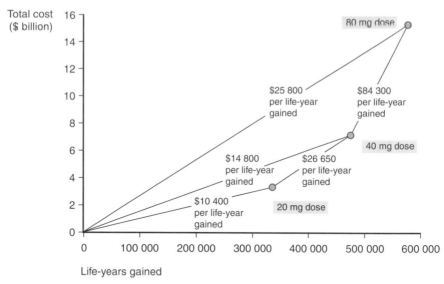

Figure 15.3   Incremental cost-effectiveness: (data from Goldman cost ($) per life-year gained for 3 doses of cholesterol-lowering therapy (data from Goldman et al 1991).

Now increasing the dose to 40 mg would alter the total cost and the total effectiveness, so that the cost per life-year saved compared to placebo would rise to $14 800 (the line from the origin to the 40 mg point), and further increasing the dose to 80 mg would change the cost-effectiveness ratio to $25 800 per life-year saved compared to placebo. However, in order to treat someone with 40 mg it is necessary to go through treatment at 20 mg per day. Consequently, the comparison should not really be between 40 mg and 0, but between 40 mg and 20 mg: that is, the incremental cost-effectiveness or change in costs as a ratio of the change in effectiveness from moving from 20 mg to 40 mg.

When we plot this line on the graph we get a somewhat different picture. The incremental cost per life-year gained of 40 mg is actually $26 650, and at the 80 mg dose reaches $84 300 per life-year saved compared to the 40 mg dose, which looks to be very much poorer value for money. So the incremental cost-effectiveness ratio is always the appropriate basis for decision-making. The 4S study cannot be criticised for not reporting such information as the trial was not designed to identify differences between doses. However, the decision-maker may still want such information.

• In reporting their results, the authors of the 4S economic evaluation gave the actual cost and effect differences as well as the cost-effectiveness ratios, but they did not report the overall magnitude of costs in relation to the size of the eligible population. As there will always be a budget constraint, the total cost of an intervention as well as the cost-effectiveness will continue to be an important piece of information.

- In looking at the sensitivity of the results to the values and assumptions used in the base case analyses, the analysts considered a number of different variables. However, this was a *one-way analysis* in which each variable was altered independently whilst the others were held constant. An alternative might have been *multi-way analyses* in which several variables were changed simultaneously.

Figure 15.4 shows how uncertainty can affect the results of cost-effectiveness studies. In case A, the black lines represent the uncertainty surrounding effectiveness and cost, and so the box is an approximation of the area of uncertainty: in theory, the actual result could be anywhere in this box. In this case the therapy is definitely more costly and more effective than the comparator – that is, it is completely within Quadrant I – but a decision-maker could not be certain that it was within the area of acceptability. In case B, the intervention is clearly more effective than the comparator, but there is considerable uncertainty as to whether the costs are higher or lower. Consequently, the intervention could be in the area of acceptability, uncertainty or rejection.

- In reaching a conclusion about the cost-effectiveness of simvastatin, the authors refer to four other studies. This is a standard procedure, and in this case there is no reason to think that the other studies chosen were unrepresentative. However, there is always the possibility that authors could carefully choose other studies in order to show their own results in a more or less favourable light. And four studies is a small number from the hundreds which are now published each year.

An alternative approach is to make reference to a larger number of studies, and allow the reader to judge whether the results are good or bad within

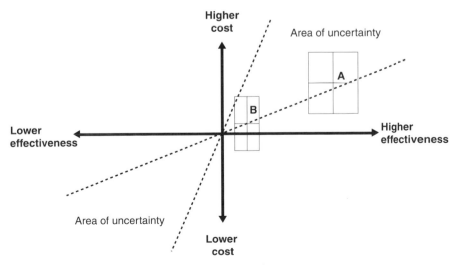

Figure 15.4 Uncertainty on the cost-effectiveness plane.

an overall distribution. For example, Figure 15.5 shows the distribution of 179 baseline incremental cost-effectiveness results extracted from published UK studies. These range across different patient groups, therapeutic categories and diagnostic/disease areas, and it should be noted that the interventions are not necessarily in routine use. It can be seen that the median value is £2911 per QALY, and the average is £26 694 (Briggs & Gray 1999). So the 4S results are probably around the median value and well below the average, and this might be a more standardised way of reporting results.

• Finally, in discussing the results, the authors refer to cost-effectiveness 'among both men and women'. However, as the results replicated in Table 15.1 show, the cost-effectiveness was actually much better for men than for women, because they were at higher risk and therefore more life-years were saved. This has undoubted distributive and possibly ethical implications, which the authors could have raised. Having said that, and given the complexity of these issues, perhaps it is not surprising that they decided to avoid comment!

A COST–UTILITY EXAMPLE

As noted above, the 4S economic evaluation we have been examining did not include quality of life as an outcome measure (although the authors did consider this hypothetically in their sensitivity analysis). So we will now look at a published cost–utility study: that is, a study where cost-effectiveness was measured in terms of the cost per QALY. Again we will consider this under the same checklist headings.

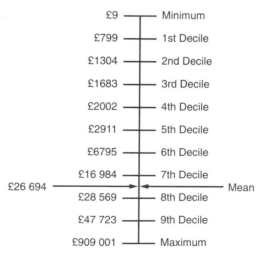

Figure 15.5 Assessing cost-effectiveness in relation to other interventions: the distribution of 179 UK cost-effectiveness results (data from Briggs & Gray 1998).

Table 15.1 Cost-effectiveness of simvastatin treatment for 5 years in 59-year-old patients with coronary heart disease and a pre-treatment total cholesterol level of 261 mg/dl

Variable	Analysis of direct costs only		Analysis of direct costs and production losses	
	Men	Women	Men	Women
Costs ($)				
Intervention	2242	2410	2242	2410
Associated morbidity	−718	−725	−1783	−1601
Net	1524	1685	459	809
Life-years gained	0.28	0.16	0.28	0.16
Cost per life-year gained ($)	5400	10 500	1600	5100

Data from Johannesson et al (1997).

Framework

The selected study (Hatziandreu 1994) is a comparison of two treatments for patients at risk of recurrent depression (specifically, 35-year-old women who have experienced two previous episodes of depression within the past 4 years. One is maintenance therapy using sertraline, one of a fairly new class of drugs called selective serotonin reuptake inhibitors, or SSRIs. The alternative treatment is episodic treatment with an older tricyclic antidepressant or TCA, dothiepin. TCAs remain the the most commonly prescribed drugs, but SSRIs are preferred by some clinicians for a variety of reasons including their non-toxicity when taken in overdose. SSRIs cost substantially more than the older classes of drugs. Depression is a major area of expenditure in the health-care system.

Data and methods

The study used a decision-analysis approach, in which the lifetime health care and social impact of the two treatments were simulated in a model. The outcome was measured in terms of QALYs. Data on resource use was obtained from the expert opinion of two physician panels with experience in the area, one containing five general practitioners and the other five psychiatrists. Data on the likelihood of recurrences of depressive illness were also derived using the expert panels, who estimated the proportion of patients on each treatment who would experience a given number of recurrences, and the timing of these. Finally, data on the quality-of-life weight attached to depression-related health states were also obtained from the panel.

To briefly explain the background to this, imagine that we can represent our best imaginable health state by the number 1, and the worst by the number 0. A 75-year-old person restored to full health following a successful hip replacement operation might expect a further 10 years of life-expectancy with no quality impairment, and this would be equivalent to 10 QALYs. Imagine now that the operation is not successful, and the person remains severely restricted in their mobility and in frequent pain. If we could say that that person's quality of life had been halved, then their remaining life-expectancy would be $(0.5 \times 10) = 5$ QALYs. Of course the precise number or weight attached to this state of health may not be 0.5, but the point for the moment is that it is indisputably less than 1.

In this study, the panel estimated that being on sertraline maintenance treatment with no recurrence of depression had a utility of 0.93, so that 1 year in that state was equivalent to 0.93 QALYs. Alternatively, a patient receiving dothiepin therapy who experienced a recurrence of major depression lasting 3 months was estimated to have a utility of 0.69 during that period.

Results

Table 15.2 gives some summary results from this study. In the base case, the lifetime costs of therapy were £3407 per patient in the sertraline group and £1648 per patient in the dothiepin group; the estimated QALYs were 14.94 per patient in the sertraline group and 14.13 per patient in the dothiepin group; and hence the incremental cost-effectiveness ratio was $(3407 - 1648)/(14.94 - 14.13) = £2172$ per QALY.

This result was then subjected to a sensitivity analysis, in which compliance, utility scores, costs and recurrence rates were varied, and Table 15.2 also reports the results of this sensitivity analysis.

Table 15.2 Cost–utility of sertraline maintenance treatment compared with dothiepin episodic treatment for patients at risk of depressive illness

	Sertraline (SSRI) maintenance treatment	Dothiepin (TCA) episodic treatment	Comparison		
	Lifetime costs	QALYs gained	Lifetime costs	QALYs gained	Incremental cost per QALY gained
Baseline	3407	14.94	1648	14.13	2172
GP utility scores	3407	14.86	1648	14.07	2227
Psychiatrist utility scores	3407	15.0	1648	14.17	2119
20% SSRI compliance	2061	14.63	1648	14.13	826
80% SSRI compliance	3625	14.94	1648	14.13	2441
100% increase in SSRI cost	4581	14.94	1648	14.13	3621
Equal recurrence rates	3980	14.60	1648	14.13	4962

SSRI, selective serotonin reuptake inhibitor.
TCA, tricyclic anti-depressant.

Data from Hatziandreu (1994).

Discussion

The authors locate their results within a table showing 12 other cost–utility results, and conclude on this basis that 'incremental cost-utility ratios for maintenance treatment compared with episodic treatment with dothiepin for high risk recurrent depressive patients appear to fall within a lower range than cost-utility ratios for treatment of severe hypertension and other common interventions such as estrogen replacement therapy or haemodialysis.'

Comments on the cost–utility example

As with the previous example, you would have to read the article carefully in order to make a full assessment of this evidence against the checklist. However, here are some points to note:

• The method used to identify, measure and value the resource consequences of the therapies was entirely dependent on two panels of five physicians. Of course, if there are no large, long-term randomised controlled trials within which such information has been collected the analyst has to use other sources of information. But it is possible that case control studies, cohort studies, observational studies or analyses of record-linked or routine data could have provided some data.

• Similarly, the results of this study are crucially dependent on the panels of physicians for the estimates of likelihood of recurrences. This is very low grade 'evidence', and a decision-maker might (should) feel uneasy about committing resources on this basis.

• Finally, the estimated quality of life weights also came from the panels. The methods section of the paper indicates that panel members 'were asked to choose between the hypothetical state and a gamble between perfect health and immediate death.' This approach is based on a standard method for estimating the value or *utility* of a health state, called the *standard gamble*.

For example, consider that you were confined to a wheel-chair and in constant mild pain, and were likely to stay in that state. You are then informed of a new surgical procedure which could restore you to full-health, but which carried a risk of death. How much of a risk of death would you be prepared to take: 5% or 10% or 15%? The answer will depend at least in part on how bad you perceive the initial health state to be: the greater the *disutility* caused by the present health state, then presumably the higher the risk you would be willing to run in order to be free of it. Thus if an individual was prepared to take a risk of 20% of death in order to be free of a particular state of ill-health, we could say that 1 year in that health state had a utility equivalent to 80% of full-health, which would equate to a QALY of 0.8.

An alternative approach, called the *time trade-off*, proceeds as follows: suppose, as above, you were in a health state which confined you to a wheel-chair in constant mild pain. You are then asked which you would prefer: 10 years in that state, or some lesser period of life in a state of full-health? That is, how much quantity of life might you be prepared to trade off to be restored to full-health. If the response was that you would give up 3 years of life to be free of the symptoms (i.e. you were indifferent between 10 years with the symptoms and 7 years free of them) then the valuation of that health state is that it is equivalent to 70% of full-health or a QALY of 0.7.

Most standard gamble and time trade-off studies find substantial variation between individuals in their valuations of particular states, and a closer look at this paper shows the same: for example, the valuations of a depressive episode treated with a TCA ranged from 0.35 to 0.95, and of a depressive episode treated with an SSRI ranged from 0.35 to 0.85. So in a sample of 10 the confidence intervals around these estimates would inevitably have been quite wide, and indeed there would be no statistically significant difference.

THE COST–BENEFIT APPROACH

So far, we have dealt with valuation of health states in non-monetary terms: for example, how much time one is prepared to trade off to be free of a state of ill-health, or how much of a gamble. And both cost-effectiveness analyses and cost-utility analyses can only answer a *relative* question: given that we want to devote a given budget to improving health (measured in life-years or QALYs), what is the most efficient way of doing so? So both approaches are concerned with efficiency, but only with what economists refer to as *technical efficiency*: how best to achieve a previously agreed objective. But of course there is a more fundamental question: is it worthwhile achieving this objective at all? Might it not be better to allocate the resources involved to some other objective altogether? This question, which concerns *allocative efficiency*, can only be answered if we can find some way of expressing all the costs and all the benefits of an action in money terms, and then seeing if the benefits outweigh the costs or the costs outweigh the benefits. This is what *cost–benefit analysis* strives to do. Although this is a widely-used term, in fact it has this quite specific meaning to economists.

How might it be possible to obtain a monetary valuation of a health state or indeed of life itself? One method is the *human capital* approach, which values survival or morbidity in terms of the value (at market prices) of the output that the person would have produced if the person had not died or been ill. Time not used in market work may also be included: for example, leisure time could be included at a market wage rate, and housework time could also be included based on the wage rate for domestic help or the opportunity wage rate: what that person could have earned. But there are many problems with this approach: first, it is difficult to value mortality and morbidity for people who have retired from the labour force; second, its theoretical basis is rather weak; and third, health clearly does not have a value only insofar as it contributes to Gross National Product. Consequently, the human capital approach is not widely used.

A second approach is based on so-called *revealed preferences*, and makes use of observed individual choices concerning risk and income. For example, it is a general empirical finding that occupations with a degree of hazard attached to them have somewhat higher wages than otherwise similar jobs which do not have that element of risk. There is in effect a trade-off which employees make between the level of risk and the higher rewards. So by observing the higher risk and the wage difference it is possible to calculate the implicit valuation which individuals place on a health state. The results of such studies are fairly consistent over time and between countries: broadly, they suggest a value of life of around £4 million (OECD 1994). Of course such valuations can only be derived under conditions of uncertainty: if you knew that the fatal accident was going to happen to you, your valuation would presumably be higher than if it was just a statistical possibility! Hence such valuations are sometimes called the value of a statistical life or VOSL.

A third method for obtaining a monetary valuation of health states is *contingent valuation* or *willingness to pay*, and is normally based on responses to hypothetical scenarios about willingness to pay to avoid certain outcomes. For example, suppose you were buying a car and could choose to have an air bag fitted at some extra cost. This would reduce the risk of death from 8 in 100 000 to 5 in 100 000. What is the most you would be prepared to pay to have the air bag fitted? If your maximum willingness to pay was £60, then your implied value of life would be ($£60/3 \times 10^{-5}$ =) £3 million. This would imply that an intervention would be acceptable if it cost less than £3 m per life saved, but would not be worthwhile if it cost more than £3 m.

This is a very simplified example, but illustrates the essential features of the cost–benefit approach. Its main virtue is that it can address the fundamental question of whether something is worth doing at all. However, there are many difficulties involved in obtaining monetary values for health outcomes, and so cost–benefit studies are currently very rare in the health field. In fact almost all the studies published under this title are no such thing, but merely a comparison of the treatment costs and the cost savings (e.g. by reducing morbidity) from a programme.

CONCLUSION: USING ECONOMIC EVALUATION IN EVIDENCE-BASED PRACTICE

In this chapter and in Chapter 10 we have looked at the rationale for the economic approach; the way in which cost-effectiveness studies should be performed; and the way in which the validity of cost-effectiveness studies should be assessed. Health economists disagree on a number of things, but there is an increasing consensus on the methods to use and the guidelines to adhere to.

Until now, clinicians and other decision-makers have used methods other than cost-effectiveness analysis to make choices about health interventions, such as guidelines and recommendations devised by professional bodies. For example, in 1980 the American College of Obstetricians and Gynecologists recommended a policy of annual smear tests for cervical cancer screening for all women from the age of 18. The same year the American Cancer Society recommended a less frequent schedule of smears if two consecutive annual tests were negative. Then in 1988 a number of professional organisations proposed a less frequent schedule of smears if three consecutive annual tests were negative, but did not suggest an alternative screening interval. However, an economic evaluation using the same evidence available to these bodies then demonstrated that the cost per year of life saved of a 4-year interval would be $10 100, but that this would increase to $184 500 at 3-year intervals, to $262 000 at 2-year intervals, and to $1 100 000 if done annually (Eddy 1992). Using this explicit information, it would seem advisable to recommend a 4-year interval and then devote the resources freed up to other activities which provided more health gain.

In conclusion, cost-effectiveness analysis is an *aid* to making decisions about health-care resources, and few economists would claim that it can be used as a complete decision-making procedure. Other values, considerations and skills will always play a part. But it does offer a powerful and explicit framework for considering information relevant to decision-making, and as the pressures on health-care systems increase, so economic evaluation is likely to become a more familiar and necessary tool.

REFERENCES

Briggs A, Gray A 1999 Handling uncertainty when performing economic evaluation of health care interventions: A structured review of published studies with special reference to the distributional form and variance of cost data. Final Report. NHS Health Technology Assessment Programme. Health Technology Assessment 1999 3(2), Southampton

Buxton M J, Drummond M F, Van Hout B A, Prince R L, Sheldon T A, Szucs T, Vray M 1997 Modelling in economic evaluation: an unavoidable fact of life [editorial]. Health Economics 6:217–227

Eddy D M 1992 Assessing health practices and designing practice policies: The explicit approach. American College of Physicians, Philadelphia

Goldman L, Weinstein M C, Goldman P A, Williams L W 1991 Cost-effectiveness of HMG-CoA reductase inhibition for primary and secondary prevention of coronary heart disease. Journal of the American Medical Association 265(9):1145–1151

Hatziandreu E J 1994 Cost utility of maintenance treatment of recurrent depression with sertraline versus episodic treatment with dothiepin. PharmacoEconomics 5:249–264

Johannesson M, Jonsson B, Kjekshus J, Olsson A G, Pedersen T R, Wedel H 1997 Cost effectiveness of simvastatin treatment to lower cholesterol levels in patients with coronary heart disease. New England Journal of Medicine 336(5):332–336

Laupacis A, Feeny D, Detsky A S, Tugwell P X 1992 How attractive does a new technology have to be to warrant adoption and utilization? Tentative guidelines for using clinical and economic evaluations. Canadian Medical Association Journal 146(4):473–481

Organisation for Economic Cooperation and Development 1994 Project and Policy Appraisal: integrating economics and the environment. OECD, Paris 4S 1994 Randomised trial of cholesterol lowering in 4444 patients with coronary heart disease: the Scandinavian Simvastatin Survival Study (4S). Lancet 344:1383–1389

FURTHER READING ON HEALTH ECONOMICS

Texts

Drummond M F, O'Brien B, Stoddart G L, Torrance G W 1997 Methods for the economic evaluation of health care programmes, 2nd edn. Oxford University Press, Oxford

Folland S, Goodman A, Stano M 1997 The economics of health and health care, 2nd edn. Prentice Hall, New Jersey

Gold M R, Siegel J E, Russell L B, Weinstein M C (eds) 1997 Cost-effectiveness in health and medicine. Oxford University Press, New York

McGuire A, Fenn P, Mayhew K 1991 Providing health care: the economics of alternative systems of finance and delivery. Oxford University Press, Oxford

Mooney G 1994 Key issues in health economics. Wheatsheaf, Brighton

Sloan F (ed) 1995 Valuing health care: costs, benefits and effectiveness of pharmaceuticals and other medical technologies. Cambridge University Press, Cambridge

General articles

Drummond M, Jefferson T for the BMJ Economic Evaluation Working Party 1996 Guidelines for authors and peer-reviewers of economic submissions to the BMJ. British Medical Journal 313:275–283

Eddy D 1990 Clinical decision making: from theory to practice. Series in Journal of the American Medical Association, 263:287–290, 877–880, 2239–2243, 2493–2505, 3077–3084; 264:389–391, 1161–1170, 1737–1739

Robinson R 1993 Economic evaluation and health care – a series. British Medical Journal 307:670–673, 726–728, 793–795, 859–862, 924–926, 994–996

Weinstein M C, Stason W 1977 Foundations of cost-effectiveness for health and medical practices. New England Journal of Medicine 296:716–721

16

Context specificity: how was the study performed?

Martin Dawes

The setting in which the study takes place has a major importance when evaluating the relevance of that research. The context includes the patient characteristics, the medical staff involved in the study delivering clinical care and the medical facilities available to them. For example, consider a research study exploring the effectiveness of intensive insulin dosage in the treatment of diabetic patients (Reichard et al 1993). This study shows the benefit of intensive insulin dosage in achieving optimum blood sugar levels. Intensive insulin therapy also reduced the incidence of diabetic eye disease and diabetic-related nervous disease over $7^1/_2$ years.

Health professionals working within primary care reading this might want to undertake a similar approach. They may institute a similar protocol, but not see the same results. In this example, the hospital doctors may have had a more enthusiastic approach to changing insulin dosage than might be the case in primary care. The professionals working in primary care may be more wary of high doses of insulin or the use of multiple insulin regimens. The Swedish patients involved in this trial may also have been more compliant than those treated by this doctor.

ON WHOM WAS THE STUDY PERFORMED?

Many studies are carried out in secondary care where the status of the patient may be quite different from primary care. Patients with osteoarthritis treated using non-steroidal anti-inflammatory drugs (NSAIDs) at orthopaedic centres may show a benefit of a particular type of therapy (Kidd & Frenzel 1996). This is a brief example of what may happen in such a study. All the patients have presented to their general practitioner with painful knees and reduced mobility. Some fail to respond to the practitioner's conventional treatment. These cases might then be referred to a hospital consultant rheumatologist. From this group of patients, volunteers would be sought for the trial. Patients are then randomly allocated to one of two NSAIDs. The two experimental treatments show a 50% improvement in arthritis. There was significant improvement in mobility and pain. The study was a well-performed randomised double blind study. Either drug might then be tried on patients in primary care but unfortunately produce less impressive results. Assuming the study had a large enough sample to be both clinically and statistically significant, what has happened?

The drug was tested on patients referred to orthopaedic consultants – *not* on all patients with painful knees in primary care. It is sometimes difficult to see how patients can be so different just because they have been referred. This difference of the characteristics of patients is extremely important in evaluating both the usefulness of a therapy and also a diagnostic or screening test. Patients usually present in primary care after the persistence of symptoms and the failure of 'over-the-counter' therapies. Yet at this stage the disease may still not be too advanced. We have to be wary about how we judge symptoms in our patients. The evidence is that we are not terribly good at matching our observation of the symptoms with those perceived by the patient (de Bock et al 1994).

WHEN WAS THE STUDY PERFORMED?

When did the study take place? The treatment of sore throats with antibiotics has been an area of considerable debate over the last 10 years. A recent meta analysis demonstrates clearly the effect of antibiotic treatment on treating streptococcal infections associated with sore throat (Del Mar 1998). This meta analysis included a study from the 1950s. It was clearly demonstrated that the use of antibiotics in patients with streptococcal infections reduced the rate of development of rheumatic fever. However, the rate of this severe disease in the Western world has reduced considerably over the last 30 years. This may be due to improved housing, social and dietary conditions. Whatever the cause, the implications for this research have now changed following this reduction in the background prevalence of the disease. Therefore this particular reason for using antibiotics in the treatment of sore throat no longer applies in some Western countries. However, in other countries it still remains a major problem as highlighted by the World Health Organization:

To date, we can assume a conservative estimate of 12 million people affected by Rheumatic Fever or Rheumatic Heart Disease with 400 000 deaths annually, and hundreds of thousands of disabled people, mainly among children and young adults. It remains a major public health problem in developing countries.

Alwan 1995

SUMMARY

It is important when considering the implementation of research findings into your own practice to consider all the changes that would need to occur to duplicate the protocol used in the study. It is therefore necessary to explore the circumstances in which the study took place. If you are considering using that therapy, can you ensure the same treatment is implemented as described in the study? Are your patients similar to those studied both in terms of disease but also general physical and social status?

REFERENCES

Alwan A (ed) 1995 Prevention and control of cardiovascular diseases. EMRO Technical
    Publications, Eastern Mediterranean series. WHO, Geneva
de Bock G, van Marwijk H, Kaptein A, Mulder J 1994 Osteoarthritis pain assessment in
    family practice. Arthritis Care Research 7:40–45
Del Mar C, Glasziou P P 1998 Antibiotics for the symptoms and complications of sore throat.
    (Cochrane Review) In: The Cochrane Library, issue 3. Update Software, Oxford
Kidd B, Frenzel W 1996 A multicenter, randomized, double blind study comparing
    lornoxicam with diclofenac in osteoarthritis. Journal of Rheumatology 23:1605–1611
Reichard P, Nilsson B, Rosenqvist U 1993 The effect of long-term intensified insulin
    treatment on the development of microvascular complications of diabetes mellitus.
    New England Journal of Medicine 329:304–309

17

Introducing change

Philip Davies

Health care in most countries is experiencing constant challenges of financial, organisational and epistemological change. The National Health Service (NHS) in the UK has tried to introduce elements of market forces into a predominantly centralised, state-run service. The American health care system has undergone a major transformation in the past decade as it has tried to meet the increasing demands made upon it, and contain its already high costs, by developing managed care through a complex combination of health maintenance organisations, personal provision organisations and state insurance provision such as Medicare. The dominance of the medical professions, and the knowledge base upon which they are based, are being questioned by other health professions, other academic disciplines and the world of business administration. Health care is in a state of seemingly constant flux.

It is in this context that evidence-based health care has flourished as a means of establishing the best evidence for health-care practice. Establishing best evidence, however, is not the same as implementing best practice, though the former does provide a basis for the latter. What is required is a process of 'transfer of information from research producers to its potential consumers' (Lomas 1993). This chapter considers this process of transfer and asks:

- What is to be changed?
- How might such change be brought about effectively and efficiently?
- How can such change be monitored and evaluated?

WHAT TO CHANGE?

Conceptual issues

Change occurs at different levels and has to be written about using different types of conceptualisation. Systems theorists (e.g. Bertalanffy 1968, Cummings 1980, Parsons 1952) use biological metaphors to suggest that change occurs to social systems (such as the health service) when they respond to the demands made upon them from outside (e.g. the government, the general public or employers) or from within (e.g. sub-systems such as hospitals, professional associations, patients' groups or carers' groups). They argue that there are self-adjusting 'boundary maintenance mechanisms' between social systems, sub-systems and the broader social and cultural system (i.e. 'society') which bring about new social arrangements and establish a new equilibrium (homeostasis). The analogy is with the way in which the human body responds to changes in one sub-system (e.g. the vascular system), or to demands that are made on it from outside (e.g atmospheric change), to adjust in ways which make the maintenance of human life viable. One limiting feature of using this metaphor or analogy for social systems is that the 'self-adjusting mechanism' of death is rarely possible, though systems theorists could argue that this accounts for the demise of cultures and societies such as the Aztecs or aboriginal groups. Systems analysis tends to be deductive and 'top down' in that it starts with a conceptual model or hypothesis of how social change occurs and then confronts the real world to see how well it fits with the model.

Another limiting feature of the systems approach is that by objectifying social mechanisms in terms of systems, sub-systems and boundaries it gives them a sense of existence and tangibility that is at best a social construction and at worst false. In doing so systems theory can deny human agency and draw attention away from the fact that it is not *systems* that act and interact to produce social order and social change, but *individuals* and groups of individuals. Consequently, an alternative conceptual approach to social change is one which gives much more attention to the actions and interactions of individuals and groups of individuals and the ideas, beliefs, values, prejudices, ideologies, traditions, fads and fancies that they bring to their actions and interactions. This approach is referred to as the *social interactionist approach* to social change. The social interactionist approach tends to be inductive, or 'bottom up', in that it starts with the actions and interactions of individuals and groups of individuals and works towards (or generates) conceptual models and explanations.

The distinction between deductive and inductive methods of inquiry is seldom as pure as the above description suggests. Systems theorists almost always have observational data (and impressionistic evidence) on human actions, interactions and agency at their disposal when they are developing conceptual models and explanatory schema. Similarly, social interactionists bring to their observations of actions and interactions ideas and conceptual models which may influence the questions they ask and structure their perceptions, observations and interpretations of so-called naturally occurring events and activities. Also, it is not wholly misplaced for systems theorists to talk about the collective actions of individuals and the consequences of human agency in terms of structures or institutions, even though this may deny, or camouflage, the very actions, interactions and agency that brought them about. Giddens (1982, 1984) uses the term *structuration* to refer to the dual, hermeneutic process whereby the so-called structures of society are created, maintained and changed by the actions and agency of individuals whilst at the same time taking on an appearance of independence from these actions and agency, thereby gaining a reified and objectified status.

For health-care practitioners, this degree of conceptual abstraction may seem irrelevant. However, unless those who are seeking to bring about health-care change are clear as to whether they are seeking to change systems or individuals and groups of individuals, and are aware of the interrelationship and interdependence between them, they are likely to fail in their endeavours simply by trying to do the wrong thing at the least appropriate level with the least chance of success.

Levels of change

So far as levels are concerned, change can take place at the macro and the micro level of health care, at the national and the local level, at the strategic level and the implementation level. The terms 'macro' and 'micro' often lack precision and specificity. Textbook and dictionary definitions refer to macro as 'long, large, large-scale' and 'any great whole', and to micro as 'small' and 'miniature' (Oxford English Dictionary 1976). The use of these terms in social science tends to refer to macro level concerns such as those involving social structures, social systems and the operation of these at the aggregate level, whereas micro level analysis focuses on the more detailed processes and procedures that underlie and make up these aggregates.

The changes to the UK NHS that were introduced by the White Papers *Working for Patients* (Department of Health 1989) and *Care in the Community* (Department of Social Security 1989), and the subsequent National Health Service and Community Care Act 1990, are examples of macro level changes which had both a national and strategic focus. At the same time, the implementation of the goals and principles of these health-care changes required local and micro level actions by health services personnel in health authorities, NHS Trusts, hospitals, wards, community care services and consulting and treatment rooms. Change at the macro level of health care, then, tends to involve whole populations, areas, regions or units, whereas changes at the micro level focus on smaller units, and the interactions and behaviour of individuals and groups of individuals within them.

Ideally, evidence-based health care would play a part at both the macro/national/strategic level and the micro/local/implementation level. Indeed, it could be argued that the 1989 changes to the organisation and running of the NHS were an attempt to make the *system* of health care in the UK, and the *individuals* who work within (and create) it, more attuned to best practice and the best available evidence of effective and efficient health care. However, the inspiration for the 1989 NHS changes was arguably more ideological than scientific (Ham 1992, Ham & Spurgeon 1993, Robinson & Le Grand 1993). Many of the underlying tenets of *Working For Patients* and *Care in the Community*, such as the virtues of market forces in health care, money following patients, and greater managerialism, represented the triumph of hope over either reason or empirical evidence of how health care works effectively and efficiently.

When introducing change to health-care practice, it is imperative that evidence-based practitioners clarify at the outset the level at which they are operating, the types of innovation that are appropriate and feasible at that level, the systems, individuals and groups that they are likely to be able to influence, as well as those they are unlikely to affect. This is consistent with the evidence of studies such as that by Davis et al (1995), and a recurrent theme of this book, that effective change is most likely to occur where it is focused on problem-solving and practice-based activities over which practitioners have some control or influence, and less likely to occur with activities that are more remote from practitioners' day-to-day concerns and responsibilities. It is also consistent with the developing notion of context-sensitive practice (Greenhalgh & Worrall 1997) and the importance of integrating the best available evidence with clinical judgment and expertise (Sackett et al 1996).

Processes and outcomes of health care

Confusion often occurs in health-care planning, organisation and change with respect to whether one is trying to influence the *process* of health care or the *outcomes* of patients and patient care.

The *process* of health care refers to how the service is organised and run, and to its throughputs over time. Typical measures of health-care process are the number of admissions and discharges to and from a hospital, ward or unit, the number of 'completed patient episodes', the amount and proportion of health professionals' time engaged in face-to-face contact (and non-contact) with patients, waiting times to be seen and to be treated by a health-care professional, and patients' satisfaction with the service provided (though not with their state of health).

The *outcome* of health care involves some notion and measure of patients' health status, such as death, survival, acute and chronic morbidity, impairment, disability and handicap, physical and social functioning, and patients' satisfaction with their state of health.

Both the processes and outcomes of health care have objective and subjective dimensions, though the objectivity of many health-care measures is uncertain and subject to variable categorisation and recording practices (Robinson & Le Grand 1993, MacBeth 1996). Moreover, there is often a lack of congruence, or consistency, between objective and subjective dimensions of health care, which means that a successful outcome from the point of view of health-care providers may not be so from the point of view of patients or their carers. Similarly, what appears to be a negative outcome of health care from a provider's point of view may be perceived as an acceptable service or state of health from the perspective of patients or carers (Davies 1996). This will be discussed further below when problems of monitoring and evaluating health-care change will be considered.

Models of health, illness and disablement

A further issue affecting what one might be trying to change comes from the different models of health, illness and disablement that are used in health care. The various disease–pathology models that are used in health care tend to focus on the signs and symptoms that are presented by patients, and the underlying disease and pathological processes that are causing them. This raises the question of whether one is trying to change the presenting signs and symptoms of disease–pathology, or the underlying disease–pathology itself (or both). The often uncertain relationship between signs, symptoms and pathology confounds problems of determining what to change and how to monitor and evaluate change of health-care status.

Wood & Bagley (1980) have argued that disease–pathology models of health and illness are inadequate because they treat disease and its signs and symptoms as an end point and ignore the *consequences* of disease–pathology for patients' overall health status. Wood & Bagley propose three distinct consequences of disease – impairment, disability and handicap – and independent systems of classifications for each (the WHO International Classification of Impairment, Disability and Handicap [ICIDH]).

Impairment refers to 'any loss or abnormality of psychological, physiological or anatomical structure or function' and is similar to the disease terms in the International Classification of Diseases in that impairments are threshold phenomena. That is to say, 'all that is involved is a judgment about whether the impairment is present or not' (Wood & Bagley 1980:14).

Disability and handicap are treated by the ICIDH as, respectively, functional and social consequences of impairments. Unlike impairments, disabilities reflect failures in accomplishment such that a *gradation* in performance is to be anticipated. Handicaps are seen by the ICIDH as the disadvantages experienced by the individual as a result of impairments and disabilities, and are based not on attributes of individuals but on the circumstances in which people are likely to find themselves. These will vary from individual to individual, and from social group to social group, and therefore have a contingent relationship to the underlying disabilities, impairments or diseases that individuals are experiencing.

In determining what one wishes to change, and how that change might be monitored, evidence-based practitioners must clarify whether they are trying to change pathology, disease, signs and symptoms, impairments, disabilities or handicap. Other indicators of health status, such as activities of daily living, social functioning, and psychological and psychiatric well being (Davies 1996) must also be considered as targets of change. Again, given that there are subjective as well as objective dimensions to each of these, and various contingent elements affecting some of them, careful and precise specification of what one is attempting to change is imperative.

Another model of health and illness is the traditional epidemiological and public health model that distinguishes between host, agent and the environment, and the interactions between them that produce different types of health status and different types of responses for health care and health policy.

By way of illustration, consider problems connected with alcohol (Davies & Walsh 1983, Moore & Gerstein 1981). If the causal mechanism is seen to be the host (the problem drinker), then the individual becomes the focus of change and clinical (treatment) and educational (health education and health promotion) responses are appropriate. If the causal mechanism is seen to be the agent (i.e. alcoholic beverage), the change process may be either the pathogens of alcoholic beverages and/or the political, social and economic arrangements affecting the availability and use of alcoholic beverages (e.g. licensing, taxation, supply and distribution).

Alternatively, or additionally, if the causal mechanism is seen to be environmental (e.g. the demands made by driving a car), then the focus of change will be public policy that deters people from driving cars (e.g. better and more frequent public transport, fail-safe ignition systems when intoxicated, designated driver arrangements), detects drivers who are intoxicated (breathalysers, lower blood alcohol concentration levels, adequate police resources), or makes cars and roads safer (air bags, absorbent crash barriers). Evidence-based practitioners should consider whether the host–agent–environment model is relevant to their practice and which element(s) they should focus on for the purpose of bringing about effective change.

The health education model provides another means of identifying the focus of change in health-care practice. This model recognises that health education attempts to influence the knowledge, attitudes and, ultimately, the behaviour of individuals and groups of individuals. The evidence on its effectiveness (Thorley 1985) suggests that it is most successful at increasing people's knowledge about health and illness, less successful about changing their attitudes, and least successful at changing their behaviour.

Increasing knowledge essentially involves information-giving and seems to be most effective when it is presented in socially and culturally appropriate ways (Thorley 1985). Changing people's attitudes requires the higher, or deeper, intellectual processes of cognitive recognition and internalisation. Changing people's behaviour also requires these cognitive functions but in addition is responsive to incentives and disincentives (i.e. deterrents) and involves learning how to manage situations and behaviours differently (contingency management). In terms of the latter, the rewards of changing behaviour must be greater than those of doing what has always been done, and must be recognised and experienced as such by the people involved.

The role of incentives and disincentives, rewards and punishments in changing behaviour will be considered below. For the present discussion it will suffice to acknowledge the different types of outcome one might wish to change with evidence-based practice, and to clarify at the outset which of the knowledge–attitudes–behaviour elements you are attempting to change.

HOW TO BRING ABOUT EFFECTIVE CHANGE

Bringing about effective change in health-care practice is not straightforward and there are no panaceas or 'magic bullets' (Oxman et al 1995) for doing so. Lomas (1993) has identified three models, or phases, of the transfer of evidence into clinical and professional practice.

First, there is the *passive diffusion model* which assumes that clinicians and other health professionals read, or hear, about research evidence and then adopt this in their practice. In the diffusion model continuing medical education (CME) is assumed to play a key role. Caution is required here given the evidence of systematic reviews, such as those by Davis et al (1995) and Oxman et al (1995), which concluded that 'widely used CME delivery methods such as conferences have little direct impact on improving professional practice' (Davis et al 1995). Moreover, the passive diffusion model assumes that practitioners undertake CME, actively seek out research information, are able to critically appraise evidence and 'make research-driven probabilistic patient care decisions' (Lomas 1993). Each of these assumptions, says Lomas, has been seriously undermined by evaluative studies of how practitioners work and how they use, or do not use, evidence (Eddy 1982, Haynes 1990, Williamson et al 1989, Winkler et al 1989). As Stocking (1992) has pointed out 'clinicians, like others, do not behave in this entirely rational, scientific way.'

A more effective way of bringing about change, and the second of Lomas's models, is the *active dissemination model*. This involves the synthesis, distillation and critical appraisal of research evidence by groups of skilled searchers, appraisers and reviewers who can separate the wheat from the chaff, formulate robust summative conclusions and actively disseminate these to health-care professionals and patients. Groups such as the Cochrane Collaboration, the NHS Centre for Reviews and Dissemination, the ACP Journal Club and the British Medical Journal provide such a service and disseminate high quality information using CD-ROM discs, the internet, journals such as Best Evidence as well as conferences, seminars and workshops.

The active dissemination model, then, is a necessary but not sufficient basis for effective change in health-care practice. Lomas suggests that 'even synthesized and accessible information is not the only source of guidance for a potential (clinical or car buying) consumer and that competition from other sources of information requires the synthesis to be actively retailed' (Lomas 1993:444). Lomas points out that health-care practitioners work within local and national environments which provide various sources of influence on actions and practice. Four key players in this model, which Lomas refers to as the *'coordinated implementation model'*, are:

- patients and community interest groups
- health-care administrators
- public policy makers (including third party payers)
- clinical policy makers (such as professional associations and disciplinary bodies).

Promoting effective change involves what Lomas calls 'product champions' from each of these groups who can prepare locally based analyses of what needs to be done and what measures need to be taken to achieve this. Evidence from successful change in health-care and educational settings (Dowd 1994, Martin 1997) suggests that this requires an environment that is genuinely collaborative, cooperative, democratic, non-hierarchic and involves all stakeholder groups. Effective leadership is essential within this democratic environment and this necessitates trust between all participants affected by the change. Adequate time and technical support to participate in shared decision-making, as well as sufficient local resources to implement the proposed change, are also required. It should be noted that many of these requirements are not present in the social organisation of health care. This will be considered further in Chapter 19.

Opinion leaders, audit and feedback and informal education

Personal contact with respected colleagues can be an important way of bringing about change (Stocking 1992), though it is imperative that these colleagues are competent in the principles and practice of identifying and critically appraising the best available evidence. Otherwise, the use of distinguished and respected colleagues to determine professional practice may involve cherished, but unproven, ways of doing things and may be highly resistant to effective change. Stocking has noted that patients are an important group for bringing about change by questioning existing practice and demanding new procedures and interventions. Stocking concludes that 'person to person contact, particularly with various givers of the message, is one of the more effective ways of changing clinical practice.' Yates & Hebblethwaite (1985) made a similar observation in their study of changing drinking and other health-related behaviour in the North-East of England, and they found that such change was most effective where it was based upon indigenous, locally based activities that were sensitive to the social and cultural environment in which they took place. Messages, media and communicators that came from outside the local culture tended to be less successful (see also Thorley 1985).

Lomas et al (1991) found that local opinion leaders were more effective than audit and feedback activities in bringing about change amongst pregnant women who had had a caesarean section and who were targeted for vaginal delivery at subsequent births. Davis et al (1995) also found that audit and feedback techniques were less effective in changing professional practice than patient-mediated interventions (e.g. patient educational materials, patient reminders), outreach visits (including academic detailing), opinion leaders and 'multifaceted activities' (i.e. more than one type of change strategy). Stocking (1992) acknowledges these findings about audit and feedback but maintains that this 'does not mean that audit in the United Kingdom cannot achieve change.' Stocking points out that Lomas and his colleagues found that change has been achieved using audit and feedback but mainly in areas such as laboratory testing, diagnostic radiology and drug prescribing, rather than with medical or surgical practice. Stocking concedes, however, that 'if audit is seen as an administrative procedure with no clear criteria about practice and no commitment to change it is unlikely to have the desired effect.' For audit to have an effect on change it is also necessary to have the appropriate clinicians, administrators, managers, fundholders and patient groups involved and part of the change process, rather than kept outside of it as passive recipients of some remote and seemingly irrelevant administrative procedure.

Opinion leaders also need to be credible individuals who are competent users of the best available evidence. They also require the skills of helping people to clearly define a problem, develop their own problem-solving skills and develop informal education activities. Educational activities are most effective when they are practice-based and problem-solving, and may be opportunistic (i.e. where they fit into existing work schedules and activities) or planned (i.e. where they are arranged for a specific learning purpose). The evidence on educational activities and teaching evidence-based practice is discussed in greater detail in Chapter 19.

Clinical guidelines

Guidelines may be considered part of the active dissemination and coordinated implementation models proposed by Lomas, though many of the thousands of guidelines published each year lack the high quality filters and standards of systematic searching and critical appraisal. It is essential, therefore, to ensure that guidelines are scientifically valid and *systematically* searched and appraised (i.e. are evidence based). Even then, there is a need for clinicians and other users of guidelines to determine whether these are clinically relevant and appropriate for the task and client group in hand.

Grimshaw & Russell (1994) have reviewed the literature on clinical guidelines and have concluded that whilst these can change clinical practice and achieve health gain 'the evidence available on the relative effectiveness of different strategies is still sparse.' They do suggest, however, 'that if guidelines are developed internally by the clinicians who are to use them few resources are needed to disseminate or implement them, whereas successful introduction of guidelines developed externally needs much more emphasis on dissemination and implementation' (Grimshaw & Russell 1994:50).

Financial incentives

The use of incentives and disincentives to bring about change in health care is well documented (Drummond 1984, Drummond & Maynard 1993, McGuire et al 1991). Put crudely, one way in which change can be brought about in health care is to pay health professionals to do it and to allow them to see the financial benefits of doing so. Conversely, one way of stopping health professionals from doing cherished, but unproven, activities is to make them financially disadvantaged to do so.

Financial incentives were an underlying feature of many of the 1989 changes to the organisation of the NHS. They were used, for instance, to get general practitioners to undertake more blood pressure monitoring and to reach target rates for immunisation. The whole rationale of the internal market, and of GP Fundholding in particular, was to shift the balance of power away from providers of health care to purchasers, and to provide the latter with the means to set priorities, shop around, negotiate contracts and, to some extent, keep any savings or surpluses that were made by good management and keen purchasing.

Providing incentives and resources, however, does not necessarily ensure best practice, especially where professional and financial independence is given to fundholders. They may, for instance, use this independence to do what they have always done, to pursue cherished activities, or respond to the demands and wishes of patients, regardless of the evidence for or against doing so. For instance, the increased provision of physiotherapy by some fundholding GPs appears to have been popular with patients as well as the GPs and Practice Managers who offer this service. As such it can be seen as an effective market response to patient demand, to GPs' preferences and to the suppliers of physiotherapy. A review of the evidence on the effectiveness of physiotherapy (Davies & Hill-Perkins 1994), however, indicated that this is mixed and does not extend to all interventions and all patient groups who receive this service. Consequently, it remains imperative that the financial resources and independence that are given to GP Fundholders, and other purchasers of health care, are matched with the best available evidence of what is most effective, with which patient groups, at attaining which outcomes and at what costs, including opportunity costs. Failure to include these factors in purchasing arrangements will lead to inappropriate and possibly ineffective services being bought, at the expense of other services and interventions that may be more cost-effective (see Chs 10 and 15).

Impediments to change

The converse of most of the factors reviewed above will normally serve to impede change in health care. Thus, unclear objectives, inappropriate means, messages, media, communicators, populations, incentives, social and cultural factors, timescales and resources will combine with top-down, externally derived, hierarchic and autocratic initiatives to work against successful and effective change. The lack of high quality, systematically searched and appraised evidence will also impede the development of best practice.

Stocking (1992) has noted that change will also be impeded if the relative advantage of introducing it is not clear, if the proposed change is incompatible with current beliefs and working practices, and if it involves knock-on effects that increase the complexity of everyday practice. Failure to see the innovation in operation (observability) and to try it out on a limited basis (trialability) will also work against the change process. It seems hard to conceive of any meaningful change that would not challenge current beliefs and working practices – that would appear to be the whole purpose of change – though clearly there is an evolutionary–revolutionary balance to be worked out that will not alienate key players and motivate them to obstruct any change whatsoever. This is where the observability, trialability and demonstrable relative advantage may be crucial to the change process, and this requires careful and appropriate monitoring and evaluation of the proposed change.

MONITORING AND EVALUATING CHANGE

Perhaps the most important principle of monitoring and evaluating change is that it is seen as an integral part of the change process and is not an optional extra. As such, it must be considered and planned at the outset of the change process and *before* any change is initiated. Consequently, many of the factors considered in this chapter should be made explicit and considered carefully before changes are introduced so that a clear change strategy is developed and the variables to be monitored are known ahead of time. This might include the following:

- What do you want to change?
- What do you hope to achieve by the proposed change?
- Over what timescale?
- At what cost (i.e. what resources will be involved)?
- Is there any evidence that the proposed change has worked/not worked elsewhere?

- What is the status of that evidence and what variables/measures were used in it?
- What process and outcome measures will you use to determine whether the change has been successful?
- What other aspects of practice will be affected by the proposed change (people, resources, timetabling)?
- What other people (e.g. health professionals, patients, administrators) will be affected by the proposed change, and are they cooperative?
- What are the ethical implications of introducing the proposed change (and have these been approved by the local health-care ethics committees)?
- Do you have command of the necessary personnel, resources and timetabling of professional practice to introduce and maintain the proposed change?
- Is the proposed change feasible?

By systematically working through this checklist of questions the parameters of the monitoring process will be clearer. The methodology of the change strategy and the monitoring process will depend to some extent on the nature and scale of the change to be introduced. If the innovation is clinical, and control of the clinical process is feasible, it may be possible to undertake a randomised controlled trial. If so, the procedures for setting up and running a randomised controlled trial should be followed very carefully (see Ch. 5 and Sackett et al 1991, Gray 1997), and the advice of someone who has run a trial should be taken. Where a randomised controlled trial is not possible, other types of controlled evaluation should be considered, such as a case control study, a cohort analysis (see Ch. 7), or a matched comparisons study over time within the study population (i.e. before and after), or between different groups or populations (e.g. by comparing the trial group with a carefully matched group or population elsewhere where the innovation is not introduced). With these types of study it is important to match the samples as closely as possible on socio-demographic variables such as age, sex, ethnicity, urban–rural conditions, education and social class.

Whichever methodology is used it is essential that good baseline data are collected and that follow-up data *on the same variables* are planned and collected at some specified time. The follow-up data should be collected at a time that allows for the innovation to have had some effect, and that meets the criterion of clinical relevance and usefulness. The basic design of an ABA evaluation, where A is the initial state of affairs, B is the state of affairs after the change or intervention has been introduced, and the second A is the situation after the change or intervention has been removed and the initial state of affairs has returned, is represented graphically in Figure 17.1. In many cases it is not possible or desirable to reverse the change that has been introduced, in which case a straightforward AB design is appropriate.

	Baseline data	Follow-up data	
	(A) Before (T1)	(B) After (T2)	(A) Previous (T3)
Trial group	Data 1	Data 2	Data 3
Control group	Data 1	Data 2	Data 3

Figure 17.1 Baseline and follow-up data in an ABA research design.

The data to be collected at T1, T2 and T3 (if used) are those identified in response to the checklist of questions above and will include process and outcome (health status) measures appropriate to the innovation or practice in question, cost data (see Chs 10 and 15), and qualitative data on patients', carers', providers' and purchasers' views, experiences and evaluations of the changes that have been introduced. Data on the ethical issues raised by the innovation should also be collected.

The magnitude of the effect of the innovation can be calculated by comparing the difference between the values in Data 2 with those in Data 1 for the trial group and the difference between the values in Data 2 with those in Data 1 for the control group. The effects of other things going on in the environment where change is introduced (e.g. other innovations, technological changes, changes of personnel, other services provided and changes to budget allocations and priorities) must be carefully monitored and taken into consideration in the analysis of findings. The possible bias introduced by poor randomisation (if used), lack of matched samples at baseline or at follow-up, and refusals, non-responses and respondents lost to follow-up (e.g. moved away) must be considered and calculated where possible. The statistical and clinical significance of changes between T1 and T2 data (and T3 where collected) will need to be established, for which the assistance of a statistician (statistical significance) and professional colleagues (clinical significance) will be necessary.

Where objective and subjective data are collected it is sometimes helpful to analyse them by creating two-by-two tables as in Figure 17.2, where + refers to a concurrence between objective and subjective measures of health status (or the service provided) and − refers to disagreements between them. The clinical significance of changes in the values of Data 1 and Data 2 will require the cooperation and discussion of professional and clinical colleagues.

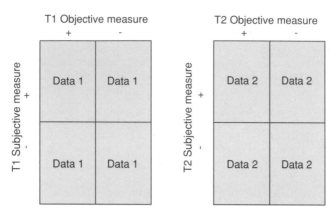

Figure 17.2 Analysing objective and subjective measures of change over time.

Gray (1997) has advised that those monitoring changes in health care should not embark on large-scale data-gathering without a rigorous review of the aims, objectives and methods of the change strategy, and not to let data gathering become an end in itself. In addition, good monitoring requires planning ahead of time for feedback of data to professional and clinical colleagues as well as to the academic community for scientific advice, interpretation and dissemination. The dissemination and publication of negative findings are as important as the reporting of positive effects of change.

CONCLUSION

Evidence-based health care provides considerable opportunities to change professional practice and to make health care more effective and efficient. In order to do so health-care practitioners need to be able to formulate a strategy for implementing and monitoring effective change. This chapter has reviewed some of the basic principles of establishing and monitoring change in health care, as well as the evidence on effective change. It concludes that both implementation and monitoring require explicit clarification at the outset of what it is you wish to change, what end state you wish to accomplish, what sorts of outcomes will be involved, which health-care systems and individuals (lay and professional) will be involved in the change and monitoring process, what costs and resources will be involved, and what organisational and administrative arrangements will need to be made. A key feature of successful and effective change is that it requires the cooperation of all people and groups that are likely to be involved, and their involvement in the planning and implementation process. Change from within is invariably more successful that that which is imposed or initiated from outside. At the same time, key people who are competent, evidence-based practitioners are required to provide leadership, act as opinion leaders, help overcome resistance to change and ensure that inertia does not set in. The monitoring of change must be seen as an integral part of the change process and not an optional extra. As such it must be part of the overall change strategy.

REFERENCES

Bertalanffy L 1968 General system theory: Foundations, development, applications. Braziller, New York
Cummings T G (ed) 1980 Systems theory for organization development. Wiley, New York.
Davies P T 1996 Sociological approaches to health outcomes. In: MacBeth HM (ed) Health outcomes reviewed: Biological, social and economic perspectives. Oxford University Press, Oxford.
Davies P T, Hill-Perkins V 1994 The Education and Training of Rehabilitation Therapists. Report to the Oxford Regional Health Authority, Oxford
Davies P T, Walsh D 1983 Alcohol problems and alcohol control in Europe. Croom Helm, London
Davis D A, Thomson M A, Oxman A D, Haynes R B 1995 Changing physician performance: a systematic review of the effect of continuing medical education strategies. Journal of the American Medical Association 274(9):700–705
Department of Health 1989 Working For Patients, White Paper. HMSO, London
Department of Social Security 1989 Care in the Community, White Paper. HMSO, London
Dowd S B 1994 Education as a strategy for allied health. Technical report. Lincoln Land Community College, Chicago, Illinois
Drummond M F 1984 Essentials of health economics. Northern Health Economics, Aberdeen
Drummond M F, Maynard A 1993 Purchasing and providing cost-effective health care. Churchill Livingstone, Edinburgh
Eddy D M 1982 Clinical policies and the quality of clinical practice. New England Journal of Medicine 296:1326–1328
Giddens A 1982 Profiles and critiques in social theory. Macmillan, London
Giddens A 1984 The constitution of society. Polity Press, Cambridge
Gray J A M 1997 Evidence-based health care: How to make health policy and management decisions. Churchill Livingstone, Edinburgh
Greenhalgh T, Worrall J G 1997 From EBM to CSM: the evolution of context-sensitive medicine, Journal of Evaluation in Clinical Practice 3(2):105–108
Grimshaw J M, Russell I T 1994 Achieving health gain through clinical guidelines: II. Ensuring guidelines change medical practice. Quality in Health Care 3:45–52
Ham C 1992 Health policy in Britain: The politics and organisation of the National Health Service. Macmillan, London
Ham C, Spurgeon P 1993 The development of the purchasing function. In: The new face of the NHS. Longman, Harlow
Haynes R B 1990 Loose connections between peer-reveiwed clinical journals and clinical practice. Annals of Internal Medicine 113:724–727
Lomas J 1993 Retailing research: increasing the role of evidence in clinical service for childbirth. The Millbank Quarterly 71(3):439–475
Lomas J, Enkin M W, Anderson G M, Hannah W J, Vadya E, Singer J 1991 Opinion leaders vs audit and feedback to implement practice guidelines: delivery after previous caesarean section. Journal of the American Medical Association 265:2202–2207
MacBeth H M (ed) 1996 Health outcomes reviewed: Biological and social aspects. Oxford University Press, Oxford
McGuire A, Fenn P, Mayhew K 1991 Providing health care: The economics of alternative systems of finance and delivery. Oxford University Press, Oxford

Martin E M 1997 Conditions that facilitate the school restructuring process. Paper presented at the Southern Educational Research Association Meetings, Austin, Texas, January 1997

Moore M, Gerstein D 1981 Alcohol and public policy: Beyond the shadow of prohibition. National Academy Press, Washington DC

Oxford English Dictionary 1976 The concise Oxford English dictionary. Oxford University Press, Oxford

Oxman A D, Thomson M A, Davis D A, Haynes R B 1995 No magic bullets: a systematic review of 102 trials of interventions to improve professional practice. Canadian Medical Association Journal 153(10):1423–1431

Parsons T 1952 The social system. Free Press, New York

Robinson R, Le Grand J 1993 Evaluating the NHS reforms. King's Fund Institute, London

Sackett D L, Haynes R B, Guyatt G H, Tugwell P 1991 Clinical epidemiology: A basic science for clinical medicine, Little, Brown, Boston

Sackett D L, Rosenberg W, Gray J M, Haynes R B, Richardson W S 1996 What evidence-based medicine is and what it is not. British Medical Journal 312:71–72

Stocking B 1992 Promoting change in clinical care. Quality in Health Care 1:56–60

Thorley A 1985 The role of mass media campaigns in alcohol health education. In: Heather N, Roberston I, Davies P T (eds) The misuse of alcohol: Current concepts and controversies. Croom Helm, London

Williamson J W, German P S, Weiss R, Skinner E A, Bowes F 1989 Health science information management in continuing education of physicians: A survey of U.S. primary care practitioners and their opinion leaders. Annals of Internal Medicine 110:151–160

Winkler J D, Berry S H, Brook R H, Kanouse D E 1989 Physicians' attitudes and information habits. In: Kanouse D E (ed) Changing medical practice through technology assessment. Health Administration Press, Ann Arbor, Michigan

Wood P, Bagley E 1980 International classification of impairment, disability and handicap. World Health Organization, Geneva

Yates F, Hebblethwaite D 1985 Using natural resources for preventing drinking problems. In: Heather N, Roberston I, Davies P T (eds) The misuse of alcohol: Current concepts and controversies. Croom Helm, London

18

Evaluating change

Martin Dawes

How do we establish that change has occurred? The process of evidence-based practice is one that requires change to be monitored. After the effort of identifying the problem, formatting the question, searching for, finding, and appraising the evidence, you do not want to leave it at that. The aim is to improve care. Clearly the question asked might have been 'Am I doing the right thing to the right people at the right time?' If the answer from your search of the literature was yes, then you could sit back, pat yourself on the back and think of answering the next question.

AUDIT

But what if you were not doing the right thing, or doing it to the wrong people, or at the wrong time? To establish this would have meant collecting the information in the first place. The very fact that you are reading this indicates that you are likely to have heard of, and to have used, audit. That is all this chapter is really about. But there really is no mileage in knowing the evidence if it is not being applied. If you have done any audit, you will already know that surprising information can be revealed during this process.

The audit cycle (Fig. 18.1) is very familiar and contains few surprises in itself; the main difficulty though is completing it. It is easy to collect the data; the hard part involves setting standards.

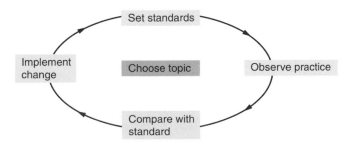

Figure 18.1 The audit cycle.

It is the collection and appraisal of the evidence that lets you set evidence-based standards that apply in your clinical situation. This requires a decision by all those involved in the application of the process to be involved. Clearly it is not going to be an effective change if the receptionists making the appointments are not made aware of the change. Take for example the implementation of a cardiac secondary prevention programme in general practice. The evidence for this programme is evaluated and the practice decides to implement a programme.

If the clinicians are agreed about the process and protocol but the practice nurses are not, then the programme is likely to fail. Many practices only book appointments up to 3 months ahead. If the cardiac prevention programme requires a 6-monthly visit, then the receptionists are likely to advise the patient to ring up at a later date to make that appointment. If that is the case, then it is equally likely that the patient will forget and the follow-up part of the programme will fail. For this reason it is important to identify each stage of the programme's process and the key individuals who are responsible for that stage. If each individual identified is involved, then the process is more likely to succeed.

To ensure that the audit is really likely to take place it needs one or two individuals to be primarily responsible for this. They will undertake to initiate the audit, collate the results, and to present it to the team on a date specified in advance when the programme was initiated. Only in this way can the team be sure that the audit will really be undertaken. So often if the task is left unallocated and no deadline date set, the audit will be relegated to the bottom of the tray and forgotten.

It is important to identify and audit all the important parts of the process. Some of these may be harder to measure than others but be more important to individual patients. For example, in the cardiac secondary prevention programme the patient's understanding of why they are taking the cholesterol-lowering drugs is as important as the fact that a prescription has been issued. The identification of the number of prescriptions issued is simply obtained from the computer system. The knowledge of the patient is much harder to determine and may require face-to-face interviews or questionnaires. The team members should therefore identify what their priorities are and audit the correct information.

The work done identifying and learning to use the tools to measure the patients' understanding of their disease or problem can be used with other disease audits.

Having collected the information the data needs to be presented back to the team. This should be the responsibility of one or two members of the team. It also requires the team to set aside a time when the results will be presented. This should be arranged at the beginning of the audit process so that there is a deadline for completion of the audit. Otherwise the process will be started and then forgotten. Worse, the people who have invested the time to prepare the audit will not have the opportunity to present their work and establish whether change needs to occur.

Finally, the process must establish whether change is needed. If change is to follow, then where in the process of care is that change going to have to occur? This question requires the whole process of care to be examined. Is it the appointment system and telephone access that hinder the patients making the appointments or is it the doctors not telling the patients about the need for further appointments?

This examination of the process needs to occur before any suggestions about how change should occur are made. It is all too easy to suggest that what is needed is an additional receptionist when in fact the process for making appointments rests more on the problem with remembering to contact the practice on the phone.

Once the process has been examined by all involved, changes to that process can be suggested. What is important is that following the implementation of the changes a review audit of the care is performed.

19

Teaching evidence-based health care

Philip Davies

If evidence-based health care has even a fraction of the importance for clinical practice, resource allocation and health care management as is claimed in this book, then there is much to be done to make known its principles and practices to as wide a population as is possible. That is to say, there is an educative function for people in the health services, allied institutions of higher education and organisations representing consumers' interests to develop effective and efficient ways for this broad group of people to learn about evidence-based practice and its potential for affecting clinical and lay behaviour.

The educative dimension of evidence-based health care can benefit from what is known about how people learn, and especially how adults learn, what barriers exist to the learning process and how these barriers might be overcome. These are the main themes of this chapter. Before we embark on a review of the evidence on adult learning and effective teaching, however, it is important to consider what constitutes evidence in educational and social science research. This will also serve to demonstrate that the knowledge base of competent health-care practitioners and users must be much broader than that of natural science, experimental design and randomised controlled trials (RCTs) alone. As important as these approaches to knowledge and understanding are, and they are very important in the quest for valid, reliable and relevant evidence, they represent only a part of the intellectual armoury that is necessary for the competent health-care practitioner and user.

EPISTEMOLOGY, METHODOLOGY AND WHAT CONSTITUTES EVIDENCE

Many health-care practitioners and users may be unfamiliar with the term *epistemology*. It refers to the study of the *bases* or *grounds* of knowledge. Since the Enlightenment of the 18th century, reason and science have dominated the basis or grounds of knowledge about the physical and social world. That is to say, for some item of knowledge to be accepted as true it must have satisfied clear and explicit standards of proof using specific lines of reasoning and scientific procedure. For Karl Popper (1959, 1965), the only acceptable lines of reasoning and scientific procedure for the natural and social sciences are those of the *hypothetico-deductive method* (sometimes referred to as the

H–D method). This is the method of inquiry that is instilled into all secondary school children whereby you formulate a question or hypothesis, which is derived or deduced from some covering law, and is then tested empirically against a set of criteria that are agreed upon beforehand. If the test results meet these criteria then the hypothesis is taken to have been proven[1] and the knowledge is accepted as valid. If the test results do not satisfy these criteria, then the hypothesis is refuted or subjected to amendment, reformulation and re-testing using the same procedures and criteria.

The H–D method of reasoning forms the basis of the scientific method, both in the natural and social sciences, and has been developed since the 18th century into the experimental and quasi-experimental method. The RCT is the archetypal experimental design, whereby the validity and reliability of knowledge are determined by randomly exposing subjects (e.g. patients or students) to either an experimental or a control set of conditions, in such a way that neither the tester nor the person being tested knows the conditions to which the subject is being exposed. It is this type of RCT that is often taken to be the gold standard of evidence-based medicine on the grounds that it deals with possibly confounding factors or variables by assuming that they will be randomly allocated to the experimental and the controlled conditions, thereby making their influence a matter of calculable chance.

The major limitations of the RCT are its impracticality for many types of activity or intervention, and the ethical problems of either exposing people in the experimental group to a potentially harmful intervention or, alternatively, making people in the control group forgo the possible advantages of the experimental intervention (Illsley 1980). Some of these problems can be overcome by quasi-experimental methods, such as studies involving matched comparisons of cases and controls, or different cohorts, that are exposed to different interventions yet are assessed by identical pre- and post-tests. These methods reduce the scientific rigour and validity that you get from the RCT and introduce confounding factors and bias whose effect cannot be confidently calculated.

The RCT is particularly difficult to use in evaluations of teaching or learning effectiveness, though its potential in education and social research has been noted (Boruch et al 1978; Oakley & Roberts 1996; Oakley 1998). Anderson (1998) notes that whilst 'the randomisation of students into educational programmes is the essence of the classical experimental design' and 'is the only method of research that can test for cause and effect relationships ... quasi-experimental methods are often essential in educational

---

[1]In fact, scientific proof consists of setting up a *null hypothesis* (e.g. that there is no significant difference between the observed phenomena or variables under investigation) and then *disproving* this null hypothesis).

research because of the ethical considerations which prevent researchers from assigning humans to different artificial treatments.' Consequently, there are few studies in the educational literature that utilise the RCT, but rather more using various quasi-experimental methods.

Experimental and quasi-experimental methods are appropriate for answering questions such as 'Does treatment (or educational method) x have a better outcome than treatment (educational method) y in terms of achieving outcome z?', and for developing knowledge and evidence about the effectiveness of different types of intervention or activity. There are other types of question, however, for which valid and reliable evidence is required in both health-care and educational research. These include questions about the strength and pattern of relationships between different variables, which are best addressed by correlational research using methods such as simple and multiple correlation, regression analysis and analysis of variance.

Other researchers are more concerned about the *processes* by which health-care and educational activities are undertaken, the *meanings* that health care or education have for different stakeholders (e.g. patients/learners, health-care professionals/teachers, executives, purchasers and governors), and the *consequences* that health-care or educational activities have upon the social and self-identity of individuals and groups of individuals. These types of question require more qualitative and 'naturalistic' research methods such as ethnography, detailed observation and face-to-face interviews. These methods are commonly found in educational research as well as health-care research and seek evidence of a more descriptive and interpretive nature than that found in experimental and quasi-experimental studies. In contrast to experimental and quasi-experimental research, naturalistic studies tend to work *inductively* from detailed observational data to hypotheses and analysis, thereby generating what Glaser & Strauss (1967) refer to as 'grounded theory'.

Yet other questions remain about the patterns and structures of inter-action, conversation and discourse by means of which both health-care and educational activities are accomplished. Such questions focus on naturally occurring interprofessional interactions, conversations and discourses, and on those that occur between professionals and patients/learners. Studies such as Button & Lee (1987), Fisher & Dundas Todd (1983), Silverman (1987) in health care and by Cazden (1988), Mehan (1977) Mehan et al (1996) and Spindler (1982) in education represent types of research and evidence from within the conversation analysis and discourse analysis tradition.

Underlying all of these questions is the ethical issue of whether or not it is right or warrantable to undertake a particular health-care intervention or some educational activity. Each of the methodological approaches mentioned above may inform these debates, but none will resolve them without additional considerations concerning the moral and ethical issues of universal versus selective action, Informed choices, resource prioritisation and the values underlying health-care and educational activity. There is a considerable literature on the ethics of research and professional practice in both the health-care (Brazier 1987, Fulford 1990, Gillon 1985, Veatch 1989, Weiss 1982) and educational (Adair et al 1985, Frankel 1987, Kimmel 1988) fields which competent practitioners need to include in their considerations of appropriate evidence for best practice.

One type of evidence that is commonly found in both health-care and educational research is that generated by meta-analysis and systematic reviews. The contribution of meta-analysis and systematic reviews to establishing evidence of best practice in health care is dealt with elsewhere in this book and in the research literature (Antman et al 1992, Chalmers et al 1989). Meta-analysis and systematic reviews have also been used in educational research following the pioneering work of Glass (Glass et al 1980). Glass's work on meta-analysis, like that of Kulik & Kulik (1989), has been described as 'a form of literature review (that) is not meant to test a hypothesis but to summarise features and outcomes of a body of research' (Bangert-Drowns 1985). Others in the educational research field (Hedges 1992, Hunter & Schmidt 1995, Rosenthal 1995) have used meta-analysis in a way that is more akin to that found in health-care research, as a way of data-pooling and 'the use of statistical methods to combine the results of independent empirical research studies' (Hedges 1992). Meta-analysis in educational research has the same problems as in health-care research, including the comparability of different samples, research designs, outcome and process measures, confounding factors and bias, and the attributable effect of the intervention(s) being assessed. As Preiss (1988) points out 'the researcher will have several options when cumulating empirical studies and readers will have questions regarding judgment calls made during meta-analysis.'

A review article on research methods in American educational research (Elmore & Woehlke 1996) has concluded that 'results are consistent with those of other studies in that the most commonly used methods were ANOVA and ANCOVA, multiple regression, bivariate correlation, descriptive statistics, multivariate analysis, non parametric statistics and t-tests. The major difference in current methodology is the increase in the use of qualitative methods.' The journals reviewed by Elmore & Woehlke represent the more positivistic tradition of American educational research. Other journals, such as the Harvard Educational Review, Anthropology and Education Quarterly, Qualitative Studies in Education, Social Psychology of Education and Linguistics and Education have a tradition of publishing more qualitative research, and the proliferation of articles using qualitative methods and discourse analysis confirms the increase in these types of research in the educational field. This trend is also evident in educational research literature in the UK.

HOW ADULTS LEARN

For the most part teaching the principles and practices of evidence-based health care involves the teaching of, and learning by, adults. Our knowledge of how adults learn has been enhanced by the theoretical and empirical work of what is sometimes called the *'constructivist' school of learning*, as well as by empirical evidence from the educational and evidence-based health-care literature. The constructivist school of learning refers to those writers who propose, and in some cases have demonstrated empirically, that individuals do not learn by the passive association of ideas and symbols, or responses to stimuli, but by actively constructing knowledge and understanding in and through their daily activities. Central to the constructivist school of learning is the role of problem solving. This suggests that learning occurs most effectively when it takes place in the context of solving a problem, or finding a solution to a situation, that is of immediate relevance to the needs and interest of the learner. A further principle of learning by problem solving, or problem-based learning as it is often known, is that the acquisition of new knowledge requires the activation of prior knowledge. Furthermore, knowledge is said to be best remembered in the context in which it is learned. Consequently, the role of experience is very important in how adults, and children, learn.

The work of Piaget, Bruner and Dewey have been instrumental in the constructivist school of learning.

Jean Piaget (1926, 1952, 1964, 1970, 1977) argued from empirical observations that babies and children learn developmentally through their daily interactions with others and their environment. For Piaget, learning and conceptual thinking arise from trial and error and are achieved by children's manipulation of their everyday overt activities. Piaget referred to this as learning by developing a 'logic in action', a development which takes the infant from the sensorimotor stage to the stage of concrete operations and finally on to the stage of formal operations. A hallmark of the conceptual abstraction that is possible in the latter two stages is the ability to transfer learning from one situation to another and to carry out reversible mental actions (i.e. go back and start again). The cognitive abilities of transfer and reversibility are important elements of how adults learn.

Jerome Bruner (1961a) argued that 'the first object of learning is that it should serve us in the future' and that this involves the transfer of underlying principles and attitudes already learned. Consequently, Bruner also stressed the importance of individuals' experience in the process of learning. Bruner (1961b, 1966) contrasted hypothetical learning with expository learning and argued that the former leads to learners engaging in acts of discovery.

In expository learning the decisions concerning the mode and pace and style of exposition are principally determined by the teacher as expositor; the student is the listener ... In the hypothetical mode, the teacher and the student are in a more cooperative position ... The student is not a bench-bound listener, but is taking part in the formulation and at times may play the principal role in it.

Bruner 1961:126, cited in Knowles 1990:91

The importance of learning as an active, participatory process, in which the existing knowledge and prior experience of learners are fully utilised, was also central to the educational philosophy of John Dewey (1938). In his book *Experience and Education*, Dewey argued that individuals learn from their own needs and interests, rather than by the imposition of knowledge from above. For Dewey, learning should be a 'free activity' in the sense that it necessitates free inquiry and discipline from within the learner rather than external discipline from the teacher or elsewhere.

Self-directed learning

This principle underlies what is more commonly referred to as self-directed learning. Self-directed learning does not mean, or imply, an unstructured, laissez-faire, or disorganised approach to learning, but does mean that learners should be able to take responsibility for their own learning, its direction, and its relevance to their everyday lives, needs and interests. Self-directed learning is often, if not usually, undertaken with the guidance of a teacher or fellow-learner who provides a 'scaffolding' (Vygotsky 1978) to the learner until full understanding and self-direction is achieved. Indeed, the term scaffolding is used by Vygotsky to refer to the support a teacher provides a learner to perform a task.

There are other construction metaphors that are used by Vygotsky, such as 'bridging' and 'structure', to express the support that learners often need in order to develop independent problem solving, as opposed to the guided problem solving of others. Scaffolding is an attractive metaphor for learning in that it connotes a temporary structure or support that is provided by the teacher during the learning process and the transfer of responsibility from what Vygotsky calls 'other regulation' to 'self-regulation'. Once the latter state has been reached, the 'scaffolding' can be removed and the learner is able to operate on his or her own. The gap between what a learner can do alone, and what he or she can do only with the support of a teacher, is referred to by Vygotsky as the 'zone of proximal development' and by others (e.g. Newman et al 1989) as the 'construction zone'. There is a considerable literature on scaffolding and the zone of proximal development, much of it using other terms such as 'cognitive apprenticeship' (Collins et al 1989), 'guided participation' (Rogoff 1990), 'reciprocal teaching' (Brown & Campione 1990), 'assisted performance' (Tharp & Gallimore 1991), 'appropriation' (Newman et al 1989) and 'contingent learning' (Wood 1991, Wood & Wood 1996).

Despite the attraction of scaffolding as a metaphor, there are some real limitations on its use and effectiveness in teaching. Hobsbaum et al (1996) have noted that in the context of language recovery programmes for young learners 'scaffolding can take place only in one-to-one teaching situations because contingent responding requires a detailed understanding of the learner's history, the immediate task and the teaching strategies needed to move on.' Tharp & Gallimore (1991) have also noted that 'with large classrooms it is difficult for teachers to know all the children well and so provide the sensitive and accurate assistance that challenges but does not upset the learners.' Mehan et al (1996), however, talk of 'institutional scaffolds' which provide structural and interactional supports to hitherto underachieving students in order to develop an academic identity and build bridges between high school and college. This involves what Mehan et al refer to as 'social scaffolding' to refer to the 'engineering of instructional tasks so that students develop their own competencies through interactions with more capable peers or experts ... groups of students are learning about school culture, assisted by *groups* of experts or more capable peers' (Mehan et al 1996:78–79). This was especially important for Mehan et al in the context of 'untracking' low-achieving students in American schools and preparing them for college education. Its relevance for adults, including health professionals learning the principles and practices of evidence-based health care, is no less significant given the diversity of professional and disciplinary backgrounds within health services and the varying degrees of knowledge and experience of evidence-based practice.

Democratic approach to learning

Another principle that runs through the constructivist school of learning is that effective learning takes place in democratic environments. This usually refers to structures and environments of learning that are egalitarian, non-hierarchic and non-authoritarian. This is not to deny differentials in the knowledge or skills of teachers and learners but does deny that such differentials warrant a paternalistic, top-down model of learning in which the teacher is active and the learner passive. A democratic approach to learning also acknowledges that learning is a two-way process between teacher and learner and that there is a 'parity of esteem' between them. The notion of definitive knowledge being handed down by the teacher to the learner is antithetical to a democratic conception of learning. The term 'fellow learners' is sometimes used to express the ideal of a democratic relationship between teacher and learner.

There is a further dimension to a democratic model of learning, expressed most explicitly in the work of John Dewey (1938), which is that teaching and learning should involve the preparation of learners for their active participation as citizens in the democratic business of the State. This requires education to go beyond merely teaching instrumental knowledge and skills for the demands of the workplace, or the everyday environments of learners, and to develop critical thinking and analytical ability.

Andragogical model of learning

The principles of the constructivist school of learning have been drawn upon, and expressed most eloquently, in the work of Malcolm Knowles (1990) on *The Adult Learner*. Knowles offers an andragogical model of learning (a theory of adult learning) in contrast to a pedagogical model (the teaching of children). Knowles characterises the latter as a model that 'assigns to the teacher full responsibility for making all decisions about what will be learned, how it will be learned, when it will be learned, and if it has been learned. It is teacher-directed learning, leaving to the learner only the submissive role of following a teacher's instructions.' By way of contrast, Knowles argues that adult learning is driven by the need to know (purposive behaviour), the learner's self-concept (self-direction), the learner's experience (what they bring to learning), a readiness to learn (developmental appropriateness), an orientation to learning (task-centred or problem-based learning) and by motivation. Knowles acknowledges his indebtedness to the earlier writing of Eduard C. Lindeman (1926) who offered the following model of adult learning:

In short, my conception of adult education is this: a cooperative venture in non-authoritarian, informal learning, the chief purpose of which is to discover the meaning of experience; a quest of the mind which digs down to the roots of the preconceptions which formulate our conduct; a technique of learning for adults which makes education coterminous with life and hence elevates living itself to the level of adventurous experiment.

Lindeman 1926:166

The contrast that Knowles makes between an andragogical and a pedagogical model of education is rather too polemic, and he acknowledges that during the 1970s 'a number of teachers in elementary and secondary schools and colleges reported to me that they were experimenting with applying the andragogical model and that children and youths seemed to learn better in many circumstances when some features of the andragogical model were applied' (Knowles 1990:63). Certainly, those aspects of primary and secondary education in the National Curriculum for England and Wales that involve project work, problem solving, students' directed activities and coursework assessment (as opposed to examinations) conform to the andragogical model of learning promoted so effectively by Knowles. They are also manifestations of the constructivist approach to learning by children and young people.

Knowles also adds that 'in practice ... educators now have the responsibility to check out which assumptions are realistic in a given situation [and that] if a pedagogical assumption is realistic for a particular learner in regard to a particular learning goal, then a pedagogical strategy is appropriate, at least as a starting point' (Knowles 1990). This provides Knowles with the warrant to approve of didactic instruction in situations where the 'learners are indeed dependent, when they have had no experience with a content area, when they do not understand the relevance of a content area to their life tasks or problems, when they need to accumulate a given body of subject matter in order to accomplish a required performance, and when they feel no internal need to learn that content' (Knowles 1990). The complementary role of didactic instruction and participatory learning has been documented in a review of 19 experimental studies of explicit teaching and reciprocal teaching by Rosenshine & Meister (1991).

TEACHING AND LEARNING IN HEALTH CARE

The principles of the constructivist approach to learning, and of adult learning, have been applied in various health-care education settings. Bruhn (1992) has advocated problem-based learning as a means of educating health practitioners for the future, and has characterised this approach in terms of:

- curricular organisation around problems rather than disciplines
- an integrated curriculum rather than one separated into clinical and theoretical components
- an inherent emphasis on cognitive skills as well as on knowledge.

Bruhn goes on to suggest that 'long-term advocates of PBL [problem-based learning] stress that it is the only known method for preparing future professionals to be able to adapt to change, learning how to reason critically, enabling a holistic approach to health, and attaining integrated, cumulative learning.'

There is a very large literature on problem-based learning in health care, of which only a small part can be cited here (Barrows & Mitchell 1975, Barrows & Tamblyn 1976, 1977, Hollis 1991, Neufeld et al 1981, Neufeld & Chong 1984, Norman et al 1985, Norman et al 1990, Norman & Schmidt 1992, Premi 1988, Schmidt 1983, 1993, Verma et al 1988). Much of this is associated with, and has been developed by, the Faculty of Health Sciences at McMaster University, Canada for the education and training of doctors, nurses and, more recently, physiotherapists and occupational therapists. The education and training courses for these professions are distinct and separate but they share common goals and an educational approach built around self-directed and problem-based learning. The learning methods consist of problem-based tutorials, clinical skills laboratories, inquiry seminars, clinical education, independent study and interprofessional education.

The Curriculum Guide for the Bachelor of Health Sciences Degree Programmes in Occupational Therapy and Physiotherapy at McMaster University suggests that:

the more active they [students] are in determining their own needs and learning goals, the more effective their learning is likely to be. Within broad guidelines, students should determine their own learning needs, how they will best set and achieve objectives to address those needs, how to select learning resources, and whether their learning needs have been met.

The McMaster Curriculum Guide goes on to point out that:

although the programmes stress the importance of self-directed learning, it should be noted that this is not a self-paced programme. Attendance and participation in tutorials, laboratories and inquiry seminars is required. It is necessary to demonstrate by self, peer and faculty evaluation that satisfactory progress has been achieved.

The problem-based learning is centred around:

a variety of problems carefully designed and selected for each curriculum block. These problems may be used in tutorials, clinical skills laboratories, inquiry seminars or clinical education. The problem scenarios promote the exploration of the underlying biological, physiological, behavioural and environmental determinants of health and the role of health care professionals. The problem scenarios also require the integration of previous learning with the acquisition of new knowledge, skills and attitudes. The problems are designed to provide a context that resembles future professional contexts as closely as possible. Problem-based learning incorporates self-directed learning, clinical reasoning and critical appraisal of related literature.

Problem-based, self-directed learning is also used elsewhere in the world. Jacobs & Lyons (1992) have reported the use of problem-based, self-directed learning in the training of occupational therapists in Newcastle, New South Wales, Australia. Students develop problem-solving skills and 'an attitude to therapy which encourages them to focus on each client as an individual, living and working within their specific environment.' The authors add that 'the reductionist view of intervention does not seem to be compatible with the self-directed, problem-based approach to learning.'

Titchen (1985, 1987a, 1987b, 1992) has proposed a greater role for problem-based learning in the development of continuing education activities for physiotherapists, and in the multidisciplinary training of health professionals in the UK. Some aspects of problem-based, self-directed learning have been incorporated into the training of health-care professionals in the UK, mainly in connection with clinical practice and skills' development modules. The use of learning contracts in the training of nurses and other health professionals in the UK is another way in which the principles of constructivist and adult learning are being used in health-care education and training.

The Master's Programme in Evidence-Based Health Care at the University of Oxford is built around students bringing clinical problems to the course for which they are supported in self-directed learning to find and appraise the best available evidence. Where there is no such evidence, or the evidence that exists is of questionable validity, reliability or quality, students learn the principles and practices of research design, biostatistics and research protocol development in order that they can *establish* such evidence. Teaching and learning on the Oxford Master's Programme includes some didactic lectures and plenary sessions, in which students are encouraged to be questioning, interactive and participatory, as well as small-group learning, private study and personal tutorials.

There is some evidence that medical students graduating from problem-based, self-directed undergraduate education achieve better professional competence than students from more traditional, discipline-based education and training (Barrows et al 1982, Friedman et al 1990, Neufeld 1985, Patel et al 1991, Shin et al 1993, Woodward et al 1990).

Shin et al (1993) undertook a retrospective comparative analysis of family practitioners trained between 1974 and 1985 at McMaster University (using andragogical principles and methods of learning) and at the University of Toronto (using more didactic methods of instruction and traditional discipline-based and subject-based methods of learning). The study examined these family practitioners' knowledge of hypertension and its management, especially their familiarity with, and use of, up-to-date, evidence-based best practice for the management of high blood pressure. The authors found that doctors trained at McMaster University had significantly greater overall clinical knowledge of hypertension and of the most effective treatments for the condition. They also had significantly greater knowledge of the evidence concerning successful approaches to patient compliance with treatment. A multivariate analysis of possible factors that might have accounted for these differences suggested that the medical school attended by these doctors was the only statistically significant variable. Shin et al (1993) concluded that medical training based on self-directed learning and problem-based learning was superior than more traditional approaches in the development of *these* skills and tasks (though not necessarily others).

This last caveat is important, because there is little, if any, evidence that self-directed and problem-based methods of learning are invariably better than other methods, or for all types of learning. Norman & Schmidt (1992), in reviewing the evidence on problem-based learning, concluded that:

1) there is no evidence that PBL [problem-based learning] curricula result in any improvement in general, content-free problem solving skills; 2) learning in a PBL format may initially reduce levels of learning but may foster, over periods of up to several years, increased retention of knowledge; 3) some preliminary evidence suggests that PBL curricula may enhance both transfer of concepts to new problems and integration of basic science concepts into clinical problems; 4) PBL enhances intrinsic interest in the subject matter; and 5) PBL appears to enhance self-directed learning skills, and this enhancement may be maintained.

EFFECTIVE TEACHING STRATEGIES

The principles of adult learning reviewed above have clear implications for effective teaching methods. The effective teaching of adults (and of children) requires the teacher to be a facilitator of learning rather than simply a provider of information, knowledge and skills. Knowles (1990) has identified 16 principles of teaching, none of which mentions directly instructing the student, imparting knowledge or any other oracular activities. Rather, Knowles sees the effective teacher of adults as 'exposing students to new possibilities of self-fulfilment', 'helping each student clarify his own aspirations' and 'helping each student diagnose the gap between his aspiration and his present level of performance' (Knowles 1990:85–87). The active role of the teacher, for Knowles, is also seen as democratic and participatory. For instance, 'the teacher shares his thinking about options available in the designing of learning experiences and the selection of materials and methods, and involves the student in deciding among the options jointly.' Similarly, 'the teacher gears the presentation of his own resources to the levels of experience of his particular students' and 'the teacher helps the students to apply new learning to their experience, and thus make the learnings more meaningful and integrated' (Knowles 1990).

This underlines the point made earlier that adult and constructivist learning does *not* mean a disorganised, unstructured, laissez-faire approach to teaching. The unprepared teacher is a poor teacher and violates the central principle of democratic, non-hierarchic learning, that is, that it involves a *two-way*, contractual commitment to the learning experience. Also, as we have seen, a constructivist approach to learning does not deny a role for didactic teaching. To repeat Knowles' observation, didactic instruction may be appropriate where:

learners are indeed dependent, when they have had no experience with a content area, when they do not understand the relevance of a content area to their life tasks or problems, when they need to accumulate a given body of subject matter in order to accomplish a required performance, and when they feel no internal need to learn that content.

Knowles 1990:64

Moreover, given some of the limitations of constructivist learning where class sizes are large, or learning situations are not conducive to small group, face-to-face interaction, didactic instruction or lecturing may be appropriate. Good lecturing involves gaining familiarity with the lecture room, its acoustics, its audio-visual equipment and other teaching aids such as a whiteboard/blackboard and flip-chart. Apparently small details such as the temperature of the room and its opportunities for fresh air and air conditioning can have a major influence on the success or failure of a lecture (or small-group teaching session, or tutorial). If the lecture is part of a sequence of such talks or presentations, it is important to ensure that sufficient breaks are organised for exercise and refreshments. The good lecturer will endeavour to present the lecture in such a way that questioning and clarification from students are encouraged, without disrupting the flow of the lecture or having the presentation digress into less relevant areas.

A good lecture will have a presentational structure which has a beginning, middle and end. The first should state the aims and objectives of the lecture and should elicit from students whether these concur with, or differ from, their needs and interests. The second part should include the content of the lecture – ideas, theories, arguments, counter-arguments, data and critically appraised literature. The third part should draw the evidence of the content of the lecture together and draw a conclusion or set of conclusions, with due attention also being drawn to gaps in the current state of knowledge, uncertainty about particular aspects of data and the direction that learners might take for their own reading and inquiry.

The presentation of a lecture can be enhanced by the use of computer software packages such as Powerpoint, which is available for both PC and Macintosh computers. Word-processing software such as Word for Windows and Clarisworks (for Macintosh computers) also have good presentational packages very similar to Powerpoint. These packages prepare 35 mm and overhead slides in appropriate font sizes (minimum 18 point) for most lecture halls and teaching rooms, and in pre-formatted ways (e.g. bullet points, checklists, tables and graphs) with no more than six items of information per slide. They also allow the presenter to print off copies of the slides in reduced sizes as handouts for students. Most of these packages can be used with overhead data projectors (usually interfacing with a laptop computer) to project slides without the use of acetates, though the use of acetate slides with a conventional overhead projector is more common.

Small-group learning

Small-group work is clearly an important element of adult and constructivist learning, and includes activities such as seminars, workshops and teamwork. A small group has been defined as consisting of 'not more than twelve people interacting with each other so as to achieve a common goal' (Kendrick & Freeling 1993). A small group allows its members to learn by sharing their experiences, knowledge and skills, using the group as an experience from which to learn, becoming aware of their own attitudes, and coming to tap their own unknown potential (Schofield 1998). Successful learning in small groups depends on the size of the group, the environment in which the group is working, the duration and frequency of its meetings, the clarity of the tasks it sets itself, the leadership and dynamics of the group and the ground rules that are established by the group at the outset (Schofield 1998). Schofield, following Kendrick & Freeling (1993), suggests that the leader of a group acts as a resource to ensure that the perceptions of the group experience are shared and to allow a 'safe house' atmosphere to develop. Another role of leadership of small groups is to promote open, critical thinking. Small groups, then, are the embodiment of the constructivist principles of democratic, non-hierarchic, self-directed and problem-based learning.

The Master's Programme in Evidence-Based Health Care at the University of Oxford uses small groups for most of its learning. These groups vary in dynamics and style according to the membership of the groups, and over the course of time. Most groups start 'cold' and often require the initial guidance and direction of a course tutor. Typically, group interaction and group-learning strategies develop by the end of the first 1-week module, necessitating a less active role by the course tutors. In one cohort, a course tutor was asked to withdraw from one of the small groups because he was 'getting in the way of learning'. He was asked to be available to the group if and when the group felt it needed his assistance. This removal of the course tutor had the positive effect of allowing two of the hitherto quieter members of the group to take a more active part in the group, including taking the initiative at the whiteboard to identify the group's learning needs, the strengths and weaknesses of group members and to structure the group's learning strategy for the remainder of the week. This was seen by the group, and the expelled course tutor, as a positive development and a realisation of the principles of self-directed and problem-based group learning which are at the heart of this course.

Use of computer searches

The teaching of evidence-based health care also involves the development of students' confidence and competence in using computer-based search procedures to identify, and then critically appraise, relevant literature. On the Master's Programme at Oxford this is undertaken by a series of short presentations by course tutors about different search engines and databases, how access to these databases may be gained and how to refine search procedures effectively and efficiently. Students are then required to undertake their own data searches using MEDLINE, CINAHL, SOCIOFILE, ECONLIT, PSYCLIT, EMBASE and the Cochrane Data Base, during which they are largely self-directed in the pursuit of relevant data about a clinical problem *they* have defined. Course tutors are present in the computer teaching facility to assist and guide students if and when this is requested. Tutors, however, do not take over students' search procedures but provide guidance and direction for solving technical problems and finding the most effective and efficient ways of searching. These more technical aspects of teaching evidence-based health care, then, are also undertaken in the spirit of constructivist and adult learning outlined above.

Opportunistic and strategic learning

Opportunities for teaching evidence-based practice in health-care settings will be variable, but tend to divide into 'opportunistic' and 'strategic' possibilities. The former refer to naturally occurring, often routine, activities in health-care settings such as weekly meetings, grand rounds, research group meetings and staff meetings. These often allow the evidence-based practitioner an opportunity to present some of the principles and practices of evidence-based health care as part of the routine activities and rhythms of their workplaces. Strategic teaching opportunities refer to those that are set up by the evidence-based practitioner specifically to teach the principles, procedures and potential of evidence-based research and practice. They may take the form of seminars, workshops, lectures, searching and critical appraisal sessions and Internet web-pages and exchanges. The goal of opportunistic and strategic teaching in health-care settings is to capture and maximise the 'teachable moment' and the 'learning moment' of colleagues.

OVERCOMING RESISTANCE TO TEACHING AND LEARNING

The Evidence-Based Medicine (EBM) Working Group (1992) has identified four barriers to teaching evidence-based medicine:

1. the rudimentary skills of health professionals in critical appraisal
2. the time factor involved in critical appraisal
3. the lack of high quality evidence leading to a sense of futility in attempting evidence-based practice
4. the scepticism of colleagues towards evidence-based practice.

The EBM Working Group suggests that these problems can be ameliorated by the use of teaching and learning strategies along the lines of the constructivist and andragogical approaches reviewed above.

There are problems in the social organisation of health care, however, that work against the resolution of uncertainty, doubt and scepticism by teaching strategies alone. Dowd (1994) has suggested that for education to work as a change strategy in the health professions it must involve collaborative learning that is non-threatening and democratic, in which the teacher acts as a facilitator, and the learner must contribute to solving problems and taking part in discussion. Dowd maintains that the crucial factors are the acquisition of problem-solving skills and a belief in the values of holistic education. Martin (1997) has suggested that the conditions that facilitate successful restructuring in schools include the support from all stakeholder groups, the cooperation and trust between all personnel, the ability to deal with those who resist change, a mutual determination of what will be acceptable, adequate time and technical support, work time to participate in shared decision-making and sufficient local resources to implement change.

Many of these factors are absent in health-care settings. Health care is a largely hierarchic form of social organisation with some professions assuming dominant and superordinate positions in terms of their knowledge base, status and claims to power. Learning in many health-care settings has traditionally been top down, instructional and expository. When combined with the claims to superiority mentioned above the result is often a form of authoritarianism and professional imperialism that is highly resistant to change or democratic innovation. Under these circumstances, the mutual determination of achievable goals, and ways of reaching them, are uncommon. Moreover, despite the frequent claims to multi-professionalism and multi-disciplinary teamwork in health-care settings, this is often largely rhetorical. The social organisation of health care often resembles that of the farmyard in Orwell's *Animal Farm*: all men are equal but some are more equal than others. Even where interprofessional relationships are more democratic and egalitarian, the pressures of clinical and administrative work, as well as research, often leave little time for educational development or innovation. A further hindrance to teaching and learning in health-care settings is the often poor physical environment of hospitals and health centres, many of which lack basic resources such as vacant rooms, a whiteboard, an overhead projector or a flip chart.

These structural, environmental and interactional conditions, however, indicate the areas in which action may be necessary if effective teaching and learning are to be achieved. That is to say, the development of non-hierarchic arrangements for learning about, and implementing, evidence-based best practice would seem to be a priority for people working in the health-care sector. This might begin by identifying who the stakeholders are in a health-care setting and widening the net to include individuals and professions that have hitherto been excluded. Effective teaching and learning can be enhanced by having individuals from all levels of seniority, as well as different professions, responsible for organising workshops, seminars and journal clubs. The more that these can be based on the principles of constructivist learning outlined above such as problem solving, needs-based, democratic, experiential as well as experimental learning the more effective they are likely to be. The use of consultative techniques such as the Delphi method, the nominal group method and critical incidence analysis (Ellis 1988) can help identify common goals and consensus in how to achieve them. Finally, it is important that feedback mechanisms are developed so that teachers and learners can learn from each other about effective and ineffective ways of learning about and implementing evidence-based practice. The need to monitor and evaluate teaching and learning initiatives remains a priority in the development of effective ways of teaching evidence-based health care.

SUMMARY

This chapter has reviewed the nature of evidence in educational and social science research and suggested that this needs to be integrated with that from epidemiological and clinical research. This involves broadening the approach to knowledge and evidence from that typically associated with RCTs and experimental research design.

The evidence on how individuals learn, especially how adults learn, has also been reviewed and a constructivist approach to learning has been outlined. This has been incorporated by Knowles (1990) and others into an andragogical model of learning, the central elements of which are that adults learn best from solving problems to meet their needs and interests, by drawing upon their existing knowledge and prior experience, and in democratic, non-hierarchic and non-authoritarian environments. The problems that these principles encounter in health-care settings have also been reviewed and possible solutions have been considered.

REFERENCES

Adair J G, Dushenko T W, Lindsay R C L 1985 Ethical regulations and their impact on research practices. American Psychologist 40:59–72
Anderson G 1998 Fundamentals of educational research. The Falmer Press, London
Antman E M, Lau J, Kupelnick B et al 1992 A comparison of results of meta-analysis of randomised control trials and recommendations of clinical experts' treatments for myocardial infarction. Journal of the American Medical Association 269:240–248
Bangert-Drowns R L 1985 The meta-analysis debate. Paper presented at the Annual Meeting of the American Educational Research Association, Chicago, April 4, 1985
Barrows H S, Mitchell D L M 1975 An innovative course in undergraduate neuroscience: experiment in problem-based learning with 'problem boxes'. British Journal of Medical Education 9(4):223–230
Barrows H S, Tamblyn R 1976 An evaluation of problem-based learning in small groups utilising a simulated patient. Journal of Medical Education 51:52–54
Barrows H S, Tamblyn R 1977 The portable patient problem pack (P4): a problem based learning unit. Journal of Medical Education 52:1002–1004
Barrows H S, Norman G R, Neufeld V R, Feightner J W 1982 The clinical reasoning of randomly selected physicians in general medical practice. Clinical and Investigative Medicine 5(1):49–55.
Boruch R F, McSweeney A J, Sonderstrom E J 1978 Randomized field experiments for program planning, development and evaluation. Evaluation Quarterly 2:655–695
Brazier M 1987 Medicine, patients and the law. Penguin, Harmondsworth
Brown A L, Campione J C 1990 Communities of learning and thinking, or a context by any other name. In: Kuhn D (ed) Developmental perspectives on teaching and learning thinking skills. Karger, Basle
Bruhn J G 1992 Problem-based learning: an approach toward reforming allied health education. Journal of Allied Health 21(3):161–173
Bruner J 1961a The act of discovery. Harvard Educational Review 31:21–32.
Bruner J 1961b The process of education. Harvard University Press, Cambridge, Mass
Bruner J 1966 Toward a theory of instruction. Harvard University Press, Cambridge, Mass
Button Gand Lee J R E 1987 Talk and social organisation. Multilingual Matters, Clevedon
Cazden C B 1988 Classroom discourse. Heinemann, New York
Chalmers I, Hetherington J, Elbourne D, Keirse M J N C, Enkin M 1989 Materials and methods used in synthesising evidence to evaluate the effects of care during pregnancy.

In: Chalmers I, Enkin M, Keirse M J N C (eds) Effective care in pregnancy and childbirth. Oxford University Press, Oxford

Collins A, Brown J S, Newman S 1989 Cognitive apprenticeship: teaching the crafts of reading, writing and mathematics. In: Resnick L B (ed) Knowing, learning and instruction: Essays in honour of Robert Glaser. Erlbaum, Hillsdale, New Jersey

Dewey J 1938 Experience and education. Macmillan, New York

Dowd S B 1994 Education as a strategy for allied health. Technical report. Lincoln Land Community College, Chicago, Illinois

Ellis R (ed) 1988 Professional competence and quality assurance in the caring professions. Croom Helm, London

Elmore P B, Woehlke P L 1996 Research methods employed in 'American Educational Research Journal' 'Educational Researcher' and 'Review of Education Research' from 1978–1995. Paper presented at the Annual Meeting of the American Educational Research Association, New York, April 8, 1996

Evidence-Based Medicine Working Group 1992 Evidence-based medicine: a new approach to the practice of medicine. Journal of the American Medical Association 268(17):2420–2525

Fisher S, Dundas Todd A 1983 The social organization of doctor–patient communication. Center for Applied Linguistics, Washington DC

Frankel M S (ed) 1987 Values and ethics in organisation and human systems development: An annotated bibliography. American Association for the Advancement of Science, Washington DC

Friedman C P, de Bliek R, Norman G R et al 1990 Charting the winds of change: evaluating innovative medical curricula. Academic Medicine 65:8–14

Fulford K W M 1990 Moral theory and medical practice. Cambridge University Press, Cambridge

Gillon R 1985 Philosophical medical ethics. Wiley, New York

Glaser B, Strauss A 1967 The discovery of grounded theory: Strategies for qualitative research. Aldine, Chicago

Glass G, McGaw B, Lee Smith M 1980 Meta-analysis in social research. Sage, Beverly Hills

Hedges L V 1992 Meta-analysis. Journal of Educational Statistics 17(4):279–296

Hobsbaum A, Peters S, Sylva K 1996 Scaffolding in reading recovery. Oxford Review of Education 22(1):17–36

Hollis V 1991 Self-directed learning as a post-basic educational continuum. British Journal of Occupational Therapy 54(2):45–48

Hunter J E, Schmidt F L 1995 The impact of data-analysis methods on cumulative research knowledge: statistical significance testing, confidence intervals, and meta-analysis. Evaluation and the Health Professions 18(4):408–427

Illsley R 1980 Professional or public health? : Sociology in health and medicine. The Nuffield Provincial Hospitals Trust, London

Jacobs T, Lyons S 1992 Give me a fish and I eat today: teach me to fish and I eat for a lifetime. Australian Occupational Therapy Journal 39(1):29–32

Kendrick T, Freeling P 1993 A communication skills course for preclinical students: Evaluation of general practice based teaching using group methods. Medical Education 27(3):211–217

Kimmel A J 1988 Ethics and values in applied social research. Sage, Beverly Hills

Knowles M 1990 The adult learner: A neglected species. Gulf Publishing, Houston

Kulik J, Kulik C C 1989 Meta-analysis in education. International Journal of Educational Research 13(3):220

Lindeman E C 1926 The meaning of adult education. New Republic, New York

Martin E M 1997 Conditions that facilitate the school restructuring process. Paper presented at the Southern Educational Research Association Meetings, Austin, Texas, January, 1997

Mehan H 1977 Learning lessons. Harvard University Press, Cambridge, Mass

Mehan H, Villanueva I, Hubbard L, Lintz A 1996 Constructing school success. Cambridge University Press, Cambridge

Neufeld V R 1985 Education for capability: an example of curriculum change from medical education. Journal for Education and Training Technology 21(4):262–267

Neufeld V R, Chong J P 1984 Problem based professional education in medicine. In: Goodlad, S (ed) Education for the professions. The Society for Research into Higher Education. NFER–Nelson, Guildford

Neufeld V R, Norman G R, Feightner J W, Barrows H S 1981 Clinical problem solving by medical students: a cross sectional and longitudinal analysis. Medical Education 15:26–32

Newman D, Griffin P, Cole M 1989 The construction zone – Working for cognitive change in school. Cambridge University Press, Cambridge

Norman G R, Schmidt H G 1992 The psychological basis of problem based learning; a review of the evidence. Academic Medicine 67(9):557–565

Norman G R, Schmidt H G, Patel V I 1990 Clinical inquiry and scientific inquiry. Medical Education 24:396–399

Norman G R, Tugwell P, Feightner J W, Muzzlin L J, Jocoby L L 1985 Knowledge and clinical problem solving. Medical Education 19(5):344–356

Oakley A, Roberts H (eds) 1996 Evaluating social interventions. Barnardos, Ilford, Essex

Oakley A 1998 Experimentation in social sciences: the case of health promotion. Social Services in Health 4(2):73–88

Patel V L, Groen G J, Norman G R 1991 Effects of conventional and problem based medical curricula on problem solving. Academic Medicine 66(7):38–39

Piaget J 1926 The language and thought of the child. Kegan Paul, Trench and Trübner, London

Piaget J 1952 The origin of intelligence in the child. Routledge and Kegan Paul, London

Piaget J 1964 The early growth of logic in the child. Routledge and Kegan Paul, London

Piaget J 1970 Science of education and the psychology of the child. Viking, New York

Piaget J 1977 The development of thought: Equilibration of cognitive structures. Oxford University Press, Oxford

Popper K 1959 Logic of scientific discovery. Basic Books, New York

Popper K 1965 Conjectures and refutations: the growth of scientific knowledge. Basic Books, New York

Preiss R W 1988 Meta-analysis: A bibliography of conceptual issues and statistical methods. ERIC No. ED300411

Premi J N 1988 Problem based, self-directed continuing medical education in a group of practising family physicians. Journal of Medical Education 63:484–486

Rogoff B 1990 Apprenticeship in thinking – Cognitive developments in social context. Oxford University Press, Oxford

Rosenshine N, Meister C 1991 Reciprocal teaching: A review of nineteen empirical studies. Paper presented at the Annual Meeting of the American Educational Research Association, Chicago, April 7, 1991

Rosenthal R 1995 Interpreting and evaluating meta-analysis. Evaluation and the Health Professions 18(4):393–407

Schmidt H G 1983 Problem-based learning: rationale and description. Medical Education 17:11–16

Schmidt H G 1993 Foundations of problem-based learning: some explanatory notes. Medical Education 27:422–432

Schofield T 1998 Teaching and small groups. Lecture Notes, Module C2, Certificate in Evidence-Based Health Care, Department for Continuing Education, University of Oxford

Shin J, Haynes R B, Johnston M E 1993 Effect of problem-based, self-directed undergraduate education on lifelong learning. Canadian Medical Association Journal 148(6):969–976

Silverman D 1987 Communication and medical practice: Social relations in the clinic. Sage, London

Spindler D (ed) 1982 Doing the ethnography of schooling. Rinehart and Winston, New York

Tharp R G, Gallimore R 1991 A theory of teaching in assisted performance. In: Light P, Sheldon S, Woodhead M (eds), Learning to think. Routledge/Open University, London

Titchen A 1985 Innovative continuing education: an in-service model. Physiotherapy 71 (11):464–467

Titchen A 1987a Design and implementation of a problem-based continuing education programme: a guide for clinical physiotherapists. Physiotherapy 73(7):318–323

Titchen A 1987b Problem-based learning: the rationale for a new approach to physiotherapy continuing education. Physiotherapy 73(7):324–327

Titchen A 1992 Problem-based distance learning for health professionals. Physiotherapy 78(4):257–262

Veatch R M 1989 Medical ethics. Jones and Bartlett, London

Verma D K, Shannon H S, Muir D C F, Nieboer E, Haines A T 1988 Multidisciplinary, problem based, self-directed training in occupational health. Journal of Social and Occupational Health 38:101–104

Vygotsky L S 1978 Mind in society: The development of higher psychological process. (Translated by Cole M, John-Steiner V, Scribner S, Souberman E.) Harvard University Press, Cambridge, Mass.

Weiss B D 1982 Confidentiality expectations of patients, physicians, and medical students. Journal of the American Medical Association 247(19):2695–2697

Wood D J 1991 Aspects of teaching and learning. In: Light P, Sheldon S, Woodhead M (eds) Learning to think. Routledge/Open University, London

Wood D, Wood H 1996 Vygotsky, tutoring and learning. Oxford Review of Education 22(1):5–16

Woodward C A, Fernier B M, Cohen M, Goldsmith C 1990 Comparisons of the practice patterns of general practitioners and family physicians graduating from McMaster and Ontario Medical Schools. Teaching and Learning 2:79–88

20

Defeating unknowingness

Martin Dawes

This book was written to accompany the Master's course in Evidence-Based Health Care (EBHC) run at the University of Oxford. The tutors were continually trying to find texts that would not only illustrate the concepts of EBHC, but also provide working examples of real-life situations found in all areas of the health service. Students on the course are predominantly from the UK although we are now getting many more from abroad. This has meant that we have been studying situations involving UK health-care delivery that are very different from some other countries. However, the concepts remain the same.

The book was never meant to be a stand alone 'how to do it' text. In fact it is almost impossible to learn how to search effectively and appraise efficiently without the help of others. I would recommend therefore that having read through this book, you attend one of the many courses now available on searching and appraisal.

The fun of EBHC is the discovery of knowledge. The hard part is the implementation of that knowledge. Both are more enjoyable if the task is shared with others. Working in groups (problem-based learning) is the method we use to teach on the Master's programme. The students come from all backgrounds of the health service including management and pharmaceutical companies. They have repeatedly told us how much benefit they gained by listening to the views of other students with different perspectives on the delivery of care. The implementation of an evidence-based approach to health care requires an acceptance of the worth of the other health professionals working within your team. Their view of the outcome measures you may propose may not be the same as yours. Listening to them will help both in the design of the question as well as the implementation of that evidence.

Share the task of searching and appraising with others. Once you start questioning your practice, you will soon find yourself with too many questions to answer and not enough time to answer them. Use secondary publications like ACP Journal Club, Evidence Based Medicine and Bandolier to make the task easier. Access to knowledge remains a major problem. It still takes a long time to get to the hospital library even when you live or work within a few miles. The development of other electronic sources of information including full-text, on-line journals available over the Internet will help deal with this problem. Whilst that is being developed most medical libraries will fax you the full text of articles – for a fee.

Once you have spent time searching, appraising and implementing, it is difficult seeing that information and knowledge disappear under the mountain of new information that arrives on your desk everyday. The advent of computers heralded a new opportunity for information management. Initially, their small memory made us structure the information very carefully making it easy to find again. Paradoxically, the rapid increase in the virtual size of computers with the associated wide availability has made them now, in many cases, act like rubbish sacks. It is so easy to think of all medical knowledge being at your fingertips on a computer but with so much information where do you start? How can you remember where you (electronically) stored that piece of information about one particular aspect of clinical care? To make it easy, there are pieces of software that can help. Some of these are available from the Web (e.g. http://cebm.jr2.ox.ac.uk/docs/catbank.html).

I have a section of my computer with references that I have found that are relevant to my practice. These contain information about local conditions as well as information relevant to a wider audience about clinical conditions. It includes likelihood ratios and NNTs. This system is likely to be superseded very soon by commercially available text- and computer-based systems that allow you to have a store of NNTs, as well as waiting times for operations at your local hospital along with the fax numbers of the various departments. These systems are likely to become available through clinical management systems. So what was once evident to just a few will become widely available.

Also developing very quickly is the need to share our searches. If someone in New Zealand asks a question about the prognosis of heart failure, then the work carried out there identifying that information should be shared. Theoretically it should be possible for that New Zealand health professional to send the question and its answer to an electronic library on the Internet. It would then become accessible to any health professional with access to the Internet. While this may seem an improbable dream, the format of this database is already in place and an organisation to help run it has been formed. Quite possibly the database will be up and running before this book is in print.

There is no point in having a system with all the information on it if we are not going to ask questions about our practice. This remains the crux of all evidence-based practice.

This book opened with a quote from *All's Well That Ends Well*. Some words spoken by Malvolio in *Twelfth Night* are appropriate here:

I say, this house is as dark as ignorance, though ignorance were as dark as hell; and I say, there was never man thus abused.

To avoid this abuse we must continually seek knowledge. We must seek to confirm that what we are doing is backed up by evidence. That means a commitment to continuous questioning of what we do. Evidence-based health care is not just a current fashion. It is the means to enable you to be an efficient and competent health professional for the rest of your clinical career.

Index

Numbers in bold refer to tables or illustrations